ESSENTIALS OF NURSING FOUNDATION

ESSENTIALS OF NURSING FOUNDATION

Vimal D Moze
MSc (Nursing)
Principal
Late Dr Sau Vasudha Zade Nursing College
Chandrapur, Maharashtra, India

Foreword

Vishwas A Zade

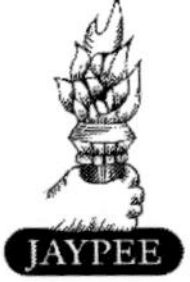

JAYPEE BROTHERS MEDICAL PUBLISHERS
The Health Sciences Publisher
New Delhi | London

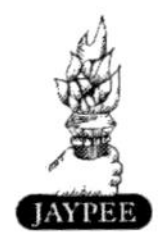

Jaypee Brothers Medical Publishers (P) Ltd

Headquarters
EMCA House, 23/23-B, Ansari Road,
Daryaganj New Delhi 110 002, India
Landline: +91-11-23272143, +91-11-23272703
+91-11-23282021, +91-11-23245672
e-mail: jaypee@jaypeebrothers.com

Corporate Office
4838/24, Ansari Road, Daryaganj
New Delhi 110 002, India
Phone: +91-11-43574357
Fax: +91-11-43574314
e-mail: jaypee@jaypeebrothers.com

Overseas Office
JP Medical Ltd.
83, Victoria Street, London, SW1H 0HW (UK)
Phone: +44-20 3170 8910
e-mail: info@jpmedpub.com

EU GPSR Authorised Representative
Logos Europe, 9 rue Nicolas Poussin 17000,
La Rochelle, France
Phone: +33 (0) 6 67 93 73 78
e-mail: contact@logoseurope.eu

Website: www.jaypeebrothers.com
Website: www.jaypeedigital.com

Inquiries for bulk sales may be solicited at: jaypee@jaypeebrothers.com

Essentials of Nursing Foundation

First Edition: 2017, Reprint: 2023, **2026**

ISBN 978-93-86261-76-2

Printed at: Samrat Offset Pvt. Ltd.

Foreword

Essentials of Nursing Foundation is concerned with concepts, principles and procedures of the subject for 1st year BSc (Nursing) and General Nursing course.

Ms Vimal D Moze has arranged the chapters in sequence of 1st year BSc (Nursing) syllabus in this book, which gives simple and easy understanding of the subject and provides guidance in day-to-day practice.

My congratulations to her for completing the project in time.

Vishwas A Zade MD
President
Jeevan Jyoti Pratishthan
Chandrapur, Maharashtra, India

Preface

Since the four-year basic BSc (Nursing) course syllabus has been revised by Indian Nursing Council, the 1st year subjects have been changed, and the need for having a simple, systematic, easy to understand and practice in nursing foundations for 1st year BSc (Nursing) was felt. In order to do so, chapters in this book are included accordingly. Subject matter is limited to essentials of nursing foundation.

I am very grateful to my teachers and the authors of numerous publications whose knowledge has been utilized in the preparation of this book.

I am happy to hand over this book to students of nursing which will be useful for them in learning various concepts, procedures and practice.

I am deeply indebted to Dr Zade for helping me complete this book and giving permission to add photographs of hospital set-up and equipment. I am also thankful to Mr Roshan Gabhane for helping in arranging pictures.

Vimal D Moze

Acknowledgments

Writing a book is a very painful experience. It took 15 years to complete the work. God helped me to find out the ways to earn my bread and butter.

I am thankful to those who helped me directly or indirectly in preparation of this book.

I thank my husband Mr DR Moze for making me aware of the potentials present in me.

I owe my parents, Late Mr Narayan Vinayak Ranade and Mrs Sushila Narayan Ranade, for bringing me in this world and providing everything for my growth and development.

I am indebted to Mr Shishir Shirqs, my elder son-in-law, who opened my eyes that there is nothing in this world like being a mother.

I am grateful to my twin daughters, Ms Suruchi Karnik and Ms Maitreyi Shiras, who were standing by me, feeding me for 20 years of my life.

I thank my younger sister, Ms Madhumati Pendse, who helped me financially.

I am also thankful to Mr Anup Dhomne, Mr Anup Gaikwad and Ms Kalpana, who relieved me of all my tensions.

I give my heartful thanks to Mr Ramchandran and Mr Sagar Meghe, who helped me earn bread; and, Mr Ajay Devgan, whose fan I am to keep me young and enthusiastic.

I give my cordial blessings to Late Mr Prabhakar Ranade, my brother; Charudatta, my son; and, Harshal, my nephew.

I thank Mr Vivek Karnik, who guided me for a hard path. I also thank Mr Gunwant Gabhane and family, without whom I could not be secure anywhere.

I give my love to my beloved grand children Soumyaa, Suryansh and Sharvani, because of whom I am alive to correct the proof.

Last but not least, I immensely feel that, I am happy to say thanks to Ms Samina Khan, who responded to my call and revitalized to put my efforts again.

Contents

CHAPTER 1

Introduction

AIM

Students know what is health and healthcare system.

OBJECTIVES

- Students understand the definition, health-illness spectrum and various levels of healthcare
- Students understand and practice healthcare approach
- Students learn maintaining health and hygiene and practice
- Students know about the healthcare delivery system, health team and roles of various health personnel and their interpersonal relationships.

CONCEPT OF HEALTH

Definition

"Health is a state of complete physical, mental and social well-being and not merely absence of disease or infirmity" (WHO 1948).

New Philosophy of Health

- Health is the fundamental human right
- Health is the essence of productive life and not the result of ever increasing expenditure on medical care
- Health is central to the concept of quality of life
- Health and its maintenance is a major social investment
- Health is worldwide social goal.

State of Physical Health

State of physical health implies the notion of perfect functioning of the body. Biological health in which every organ is in perfect harmony with rest of the body.

Signs of physical health are good complexion, a clean skin, bright eyes, lustrous hair, well-clothed body with firm flesh, not too fat, sweet breath, good appetite, sound sleep, regular activity of the bowel and bladder, and smooth and easy coordinated body movements.

Good Mental Health

Good mental health is ability to respond to the many varied experience of life with flexibility and sense of purpose.

"A state of balance between the individual and the surrounding world, a state of harmony between oneself and others, a coexistence between the realities of the self and that of other people and that of environment".

Social Health

Social health is defined as "quantity and quality of an individual's interpersonal relationship and the extent of involvement with the community. Spiritual aspect includes integrity, principles and ethics, purpose of life and commitment to some higher being.

Health Illness Continuum

Illness

At first, person perceives himself to be ill because of familiarity of symptoms or knowledge that illness is present. Then, person evaluates the degree of threat to self that the illness presents and then the action consisting of self-treatment or taking assistance or advice from others or nothing is done.

Sick person may not be able to perform expected roles and tasks normally. He is exempted from normal social roles. Being sick is undesirable and sick person wants to get well and seek technically competent help.

Disease is a condition in which body health is impaired, a departure from state of health and alteration of the human body, interrupting the program of vital functions.

Diseases may be:
- Inapparent cases—severe manifestations
- Caused by more than one organism
- Short duration or long duration.

Diseases refer to something wrong with bodily functions whereas illness refers to presence of specific disease and individual's perception and behavior in response to disease and impact of disease on psychological environment. Sickness is the state of social dysfunction.

There are different theories of diseases:

- **Germ theory:** Disease is caused by germs
- **Multifactorial causation:** Disease is due to many factors.

Social, psychological, cultural, economic, genetic factor are also equally responsible for diseases. Heredity, environment, lifestyle, socioeconomic condition, health and family welfare services, and other factors are responsible for health.

Health and disease lie along the continuum.

The lowest point on health disease spectrum is death and the highest point is positive health.

Spectrum concept of health emphasizes that health of an individual is not static. It is a process of continuous change. Person may function at maximum level of health today and diminished levels of health tomorrow.

Factors Influencing Health (Flowchart 1.1)

Age of Developmental Stage

There are different stages of development in an individual. Newborn, neonate, infant, toddler, preschooler, schooler, adolescent, adult, reproductive age, old adult, old age. Person's thoughts and behavior, changes throughout life. Newborn, under five children, women are vulnerable group. Nutrition, personal hygiene, exercise, recreation, freedom from anxiety and fear, immunization, proper care during physical and psychological changes keeps a person healthy throughout his or her life.

Flowchart 1.1: Factors influencing health

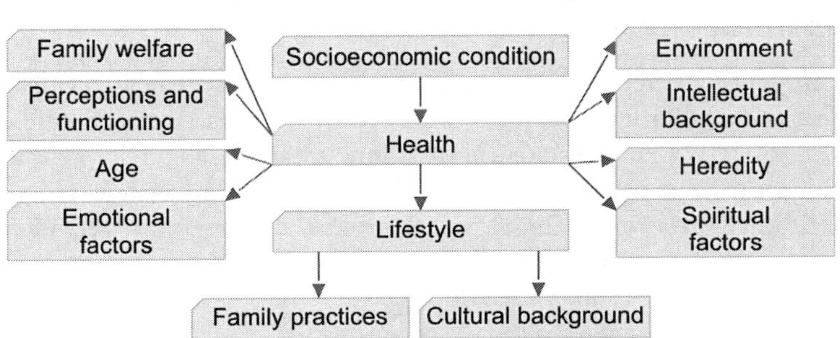

Intellectual Background

Lack of knowledge, incorrect information about body function and illness, educational background and past experiences influence on thinking of individual about his health. Cognitive ability, shape the way he/she thinks and applies knowledge of health to personal health practices.

Perception and Functioning

The way persons perceive their physical functioning affects health practices.

Emotional Factors

Persons degree of stress, depression or fear can influence health practice.

Spiritual Factors

This factor influences in a way, how a person lives his or her life and includes values and beliefs. Some religious practices may prevent a person from certain treatment.

Family Practices

Some families with wrong health practices are bound to suffer from disease, e.g. eating habits, food fads, smoking, drinking, unhygienic practices.

Socioeconomic Factors

A person who has high utility bills, a large family and low income, tends to give higher priority to food and shelter than to costly drugs and treatment or expensive food or a special diet.

Cultural Background

It influences beliefs, values, customs and approach to health care. It refers to the ability of members to plan activities that control nature or environmental factors. Biological variations are those which differentiate one group from other, e.g. body build, skin color, genetic variations, nutritional variations. Family, social groups and organizations effect environment, e.g. unemployment, homelessness, poverty. Language difference produces communication gap.

Risk Factors for Developing Illness

Risk factor is any situation, habit, social or environmental condition, physiological or psychological condition, developmental or intellectual condition that increases vulnerability of an individual or group to an illness or accident.

Age

Age increases or decreases susceptibility to certain illness. Premature infants and newborns are susceptible to infection. Risk of heart disease increases with age. Young adults are more at risk with accident. Reproductive age group women are at risk in pregnancy and delivery. Menopausal women are at risk of cancer cervix. Old age males are at risk of enlarged prostate.

Genetic and Physiological Factors

Pregnancy, obesity increases stress on physiological system. Diabetes, cancer, heart diseases, kidney diseases, mental illness, certain syndromes, blood disorders, cataract are hereditary in nature.

Environment

Air, water, soil around where we live, determines how we live, what we eat, disease agents to whom we are exposed, our state of health and the way we adapt. Person's living and working environment can influence or increase the risk for disease. Persons living near to waste disposal sites, working in chemical and other factories are at risk of developing allergies, cancer, respiratory diseases, etc. Hot climates where atmospheric temperature rises above 42°C are at risk of heatstroke, and temperature below 10°C are at risk of developing frostbite, hypothermia. Cosmopolitan cities and highways give risk to accidents. Disasters like flood, fire may occur where people stay near river or water. Landsliding is common in mountain areas. Labors and mine workers are at risk of accidents. Living in crowded, unhygienic environment keeps us at risk of skin infections, bacterial diseases. Persons with pulmonary tuberculosis may spread it in family.

Lifestyle

Activities and habits, practices, involve risk factors. Sedentary lifestyle, overeating, insufficient rest or sleep, poor personal hygiene, use of tobacco, alcohol, drug abuse, unsafe sex, multiple sex partners, sky diving, mountain climbing are some factors for risk of diseases like diabetes, heart disease, AIDS, mental illness, accidents. Stress is also a risk factor. Life-threatening illness, life events such as divorce, pregnancy, death of spouse or family member, financial instabilities, job related stress can lead to mental illness or mental overload.

BODY DEFENSE

Pathogenic organisms may enter our body through respiratory, gastrointestinal system and adhere to skin. Each system has defense mechanism that suits to its structure and function. Cilia in respiratory system protects lungs and trachea by moving mucus upwards to remove trapped organisms to pharynx. Hydrochloric acid in stomach destroy many of the organisms entering through food and water. Bile from liver also destroys some bacteria. Doderlein's bacilli maintain vaginal acid medium and prevents organisms from entering. Body's cellular response to injury or infection is inflammation. It is a vascular reaction that delivers fluid, blood products, and nutrients to the tissues in the area of injury. It neutralizes and removes dead tissues and repair process starts. Inflammatory response may be due to physical, chemical agents or microorganisms. Trauma, extreme temperature, radiation, poisons, chemicals cause reaction. Inflammatory response includes edema, phagocytosis, leukocytosis, exudate formation (serous, sanguineous, purulent), tissue repair, formation of granulation tissue and scar formation.

Immunity (Flowchart 1.2)

Immunity is resistance possessed by the body to infectious disease, foreign tissues, foreign nontoxic substances and other antigens.

Types

Humoral

It takes place in body fluids and is connected with antibody and compliment activities.

Cellular

It involves variety of activities designed to destroy or at least contain cells that are recognized by body as alian and harmful. Both types are

Flowchart 1.2: Immunity

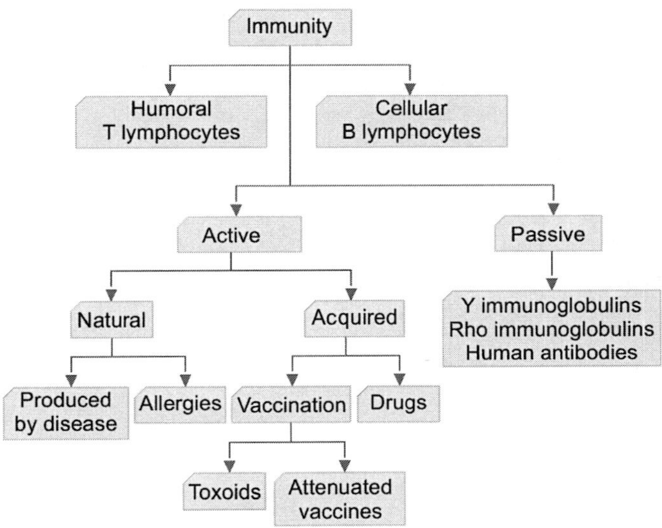

instigated by lymphocytes that originate in the bone marrow as stem cells and later are converted into mature cells having specific properties and functions. B lymphocytes mature into plasma cells which form antibodies. T lymphocytes are concerned with humoral immunity and late immune response. In active immunity, the individual produces effector units following stimulation by antigen. Natural immunity is produced by disease and environmentally-acquired allergies. Artificial immunity is produced via vaccination and allergens from therapeutic drugs. In passive immunity, individual receives effector units that are produced by an animal, another human or by genetic engineering procedures. Natural immunity is produced via colostrums and across the placenta. Artificial immunity is produced through pooled Y immune globulins, Rho (D) immune globulin and genetically engineered human antibody.

Immunizations (Table 1.1)

It is a process by which resistance to an infectious disease is produced or augmented. The act of creating immunity by artificial means. Active immunity is produced by injecting small amount of attenuated or dead

Table 1.1: Immunization schedule

Name	*Dose*	*Age*	*Method*	*Immunity against*
Oral polio	2 drops	0 months	Oral	Polio
BCG	0.1 mL	0 months	Intradermal	Tuberculosis
Oral polio	2 drops	1.5 months	Oral	Polio
DPT	0.5 mL	1.5 months	IM	Diphtheria Pertussis Tetanus
Hepatitis B	0.5 mL	1.5 months	Subcutaneous	Hepatitis B
Oral polio	2 drops	2.5–3 months	Oral	Polio
DPT	0.5 mL	2.5–3 months	IM	Diphtheria Pertussis Tetanus
Oral polio	2 drops	3.5–4 months	Oral	Polio
DPT	0.5 mL	3.5–4 months	IM	Diphtheria Pertussis Tetanus
MMR	0.5 mL	9–11 months	Subcutaneous	Measles Mumps Rubella
DPT	0.5 mL	16–24 months	IM	Diphtheria Pertussis Tetanus
DT	0.5 mL	6 years	IM	Diphtheria Tetanus
TT	0.5 mL	10 years	Subcutaneous	Tetanus
TT	0.5 mL	16 years, pregnancy	Subcutaneous	Tetanus

organisms or modified toxins into the body. It produces antibodies in body. Passive immunity or antibodies are produced by a person or animal and are introduced into person's bloodstream for protection against pathogen.

Illness and Illness Behavior

Illness is a state in which person's physical, emotional, intellectual, social, developmental and spiritual functioning is diminished or impaired. Acute illness is severe and of short duration. Chronic illness persists usually longer than 6 months. Chronic disease may disable person. People the way they act in illness, is illness behavior. It includes how they define and interpret their symptoms, remedial actions they take, healthcare system they use. Illness behaviors can be coping behaviors. It may be temporary release from role and responsibility, added stress, release from social responsibilities. If people believe that symptoms are serious and life-threatening, they seek assistance. Chronically ill people may become less involved in their care and may not comply. External variables like economic variable, accessibility to health care, social group, cultural background may affect illness behavior. Social group may assist in recognizing symptoms and support. Family, friends, coworkers all influence client's illness behavior.

Impact of Illness on Patient and Family

Each person reacts to illness differently and, therefore, nursing interventions must be individualized. Severe illness particularly life-threatening can lead to extensive emotional and behavioral changes like anxiety, shock, denial, anger, withdrawal, acknowledgment, acceptance, rehabilitation.

Impact on Body Image

It is subjective concept of physical appearance. Some diseases result in changes in body image. Loss of limb, body organ, skin changes, body weight changes, and disfigurement. When change in body image occurs person adjusts through phases of shock, withdrawal, acknowledgment, acceptance, rehabilitation.

Impact on Self-concept

Self-concept is mental self-image of strengths and weakness in all aspects of personality. It depends on body image, roles, psychology and spirituality. It is important in relationship with other family members. Due to change in self-concept, patient may not meet the family expectations and as a result, family members may change their interactions with patient.

Impact on Family Roles

People may have various roles in life like wage earner, decision maker, professional, child, sibling or parent. Change in role may be subtle and short, or drastic and long. Specific counseling and guidance is needed.

Impact on Family Dynamics

It is a process by which family functions, makes decisions, gives support, copes with changes and challenges. Illness brings about temporary or permanent change in family dynamics.

HEALTHCARE SERVICES

- Hospital-based healthcare services
- Community-based health services.

Hospital-based Healthcare Services

Emergency departments, urgent care centers, critical care units and in-patient medical, surgical units are the sites where intensive and extensive care of secondary and tertiary level are given. In these settings, nurses work with health team to plan, coordinate and deliver care to patients who are seriously ill. Nurse monitors effectiveness of care and improvement, which could be made. Nurses working in acute care units must respond attentively to the needs of patients and their satisfaction about care is major factor. Customer service is philosophy of successful acute care units. Case management and critical pathway are the methods of patient care. Intensive care units where patients are monitored closely and receive intensive medical care. These units are equipped with advanced machines and monitors, ventilators, etc. Critical care principles, methods and techniques are essential for staff working in these specialized care units. It is most expensive care. Specialized hospitals like mental hospital, cancer hospital, cath labs, renal units and general inpatient hospitals for diagnosis and treatment, surgeries, childbirths, treatment of communicable diseases, are the areas where nurses deliver health care to patients.

Community-based Health Services

Preventive and promotive health services are provided to community. Primary health care is the first approach regarding preventive health support and is used to provide health care at basic level. Rural hospitals give emergency care and transfer to higher level hospitals. Basic laboratory services, blood transfusion and X-ray facility is available. Operation theater and specialist services are provided at rural hospitals. Primary health center caters to health needs of 30,000 population. Basic health care, preventive and promotive health activities are carried out. Implementation of various national health programs like reproductive and child health (RCH), immunizations, family welfare services, prevention of communicable diseases, environmental sanitation, safe drinking water.

About 5–6 subcenters in one primary health center, serves 3,000–5,000 population. Multipurpose health worker, female and male work at subcenter level. There are also community workers from community participating in health activity.

Diagnosis, Treatment, Rehabilitation, Continuing Care

Diagnosis

Diagnosis is made on the basis of history, physical examination, laboratory investigation reports, ultrasonography, X-rays and various diagnostic tests. Provisionally, it is made on the basis of assessment and confirmed by investigations.

Treatment

Medical treatment by rest, comfort, drugs, various therapies, diet, active and passive exercises, lifesaving procedures, oxygen administration, fluid therapy, diuresis, hormonal therapy, etc. Surgical treatment by removal of organs, anastamosis, repairs, ostomies, endoscopic removals, radiation therapy, cosmetic surgeries, cardiac and other special surgeries, organ transplants and prosthesis.

Rehabilitation

It is restoration of a person to the fullest physical, mental, social, vocational and economic usefulness possible.

Patients require it after physical, mental illness, injury or chemical addiction. Making necessary changes in lifestyle, learn to function with limitations of their disease de-addiction, etc. Rehabilitation can be done in healthcare settings, outpatient departments, rehabilitation centers and home. Patients who have severe disabilities like stroke, spinal injury require long-term rehabilitation, extended care facility, skilled nursing at home with specific rehabilitation strategies so as to achieve maximum level of function and independence.

Continuing Care

Chronically ill and disabled patients need continuing care. In continuing care, health, personal and social services are provided for long-period to persons who are disabled or suffer from diseases like cancer. Old age homes, community centers, home care, hospice care are examples of continuing care.

Healthcare Team

Hospital Healthcare Team

- Physicians and surgeons, specialists
- Medical officers, casualty medical officer, resident medical officers
- Nursing superintendent, sister in charges, staff nurses, auxiliary nurse midwife (ANM)
- Laboratory technicians, X-ray technicians, maintenance staff
- Attendants, ayahs, sweepers, clerical and office staff.

Community Setup Health Team

District health officer, medical officers (one administrative), two other medical officers at primary health center, health assistants, health workers male and female, and at rural hospital medical superintendent, in charge sister, staff nurses, lab technician, X-ray technician, attendants, sweepers, driver and clerical staff.

Healthcare Agencies (Flowchart 1.3)

Public Sector

- Subcenter, primary health center
- Community health centers, rural hospitals, subdistrict hospitals, district hospitals, specialty hospitals, teaching hospitals
- Health Insurance Schemes, Employees State Insurance Scheme (ESIS), Central Government Health Scheme (CGHS)
- Defense services, railways.

Private Sector

Private hospitals, polyclinics, nursing homes and dispensaries.

Indigenous System of Medicine

Ayurveda, Siddha, Unani, Tibbi, Homeopathy, unregistered practitioners, Naturopathy.

Flowchart 1.3: Healthcare agencies

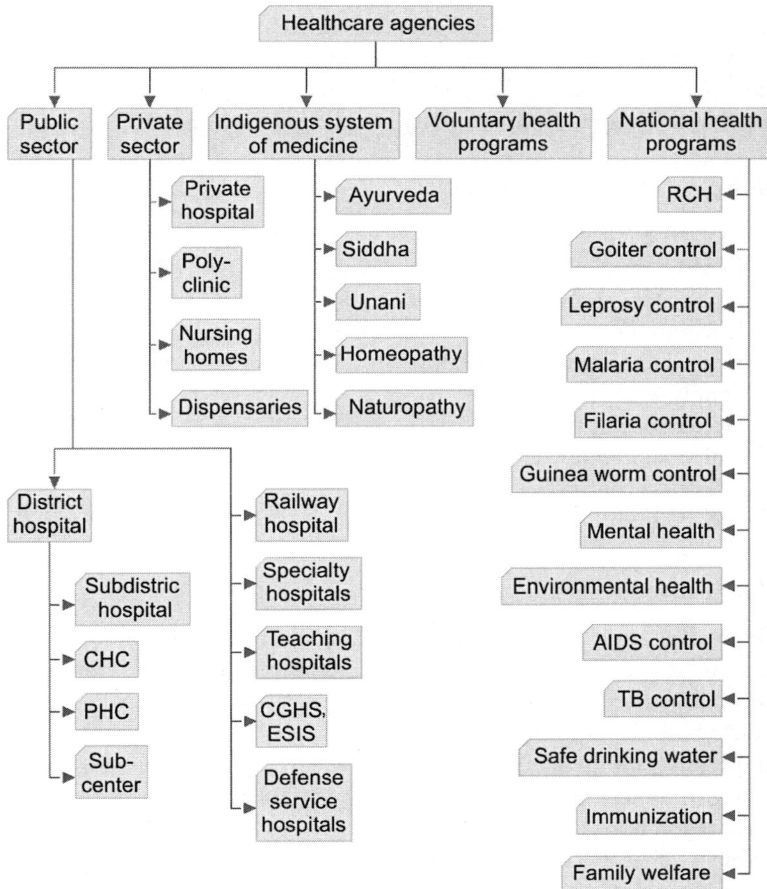

Abbreviations: CHC, community health center; PHC, primary health care; CGHS, Central Government Health Scheme; ESIS, Employees State Insurance Scheme; RCH, reproductive and child health; AIDS, acquired immunodeficiency syndrome; TB, tuberculosis

Voluntary Health Agencies

St John Ambulance, other local organizations involved in health activities like diagnostic camps, blood donation, health education. Food and Agriculture Organization (FAO), Cooperative for Assistance and Relief Everywhere (CARE), United states Agencey for International Development (USAID), Ford foundation, Rockfeller foundation, Red Cross, United Nations Development Program (UNDP), United Nations childeren's Fund (UNICEF), World Health Organization (WHO), are some of the international voluntary health agencies.

National Health Programs

- Malaria control program
- Filaria control program
- Safe water supply
- Environmental sanitation
- Reproduction and child health
- Family welfare
- Goiter control
- Universal immunization
- Blindness control
- Mental health.

Hospitals

Depending on types of patients and bed strength: General hospitals, mental hospitals, teaching hospitals, trauma care hospitals, maternity hospitals, isolation hospitals, specialty hospitals, superspecialty hospitals, cancer hospitals, sanitorium, leprosy hospitals.
Depending on ownership of hospital: Central government hospitals, state government hospitals, private hospitals, public hospitals, trust, ESIS, corporation hospitals.
Others: Subacute care facilities, home healthcare agencies, renal dialysis centers, hospice, mental hospital, emergency centers.

Hospital

Hospital is an institution for the care, diagnosis and treatment of the sick and injured. A hospital is residential establishment which provides short-term and long-term medical care consisting of observational, diagnostic, therapeutic and rehabilitative services for persons suffering or suspected to be suffering from disease or injury and parturients.

Departments

Medical and surgical units or wards, pediatric, obstetric, gynecology, orthopedic department, operation theater, outpatient department, casualty, blood bank, X-ray department, central laboratory, pathology, intensive care unit (ICU), intensive cardiac care unit (ICCU), neonatal intensive care unit (NICU), mortuary, clinics—antenatal clinic, postnatal clinic, family welfare clinic, under 5 clinic.

Medical record department, maintenance department, kitchen, central sterile supply department (CSSD), nursing department and establishment.

Functions

Curative Treatment and Providing Therapeutic Environment

Hospitals provide therapeutic environment for rest, comfort, diagnostic procedures, medications and treatment, surgery to cure the various diseases. Life saving measures through skilled personnel, e.g. cardiopulmonary resuscitation (CPR), blood transfusion, IV infusions, tracheostomy, venesection, defibrillation, ventilation, etc.

Specialized Treatments

Specialized surgeries and other treatments like intensive care, cancer care, chemotherapy, kidney and heart transplants, prosthesis and transplants, plastic surgery, laser surgery, dialysis, neurosurgery, trauma care.

Preventive Services

Services to prevent communicable diseases, prevention of complications and early diagnosis through Pap smear, health check-up, immunizations, treatment of anemia, nutritional supplements, vitamin A solution, etc.

Rehabilitative Services

Physiotherapies and occupational therapies, reconstructive surgeries, and social services.

Education and Research

Teaching hospitals provide medical education, nursing education, clinical field for the practice and medical record.

HEALTH PROMOTION AND LEVELS OF DISEASE PREVENTION

There are four levels of disease prevention.

1. Primordial prevention
2. Primary prevention
3. Secondary prevention
4. Tertiary prevention.

Primordial Prevention

It is prevention of the development of risk factors in population in which they have not yet appeared, e.g. obesity, hypertension have their origin in childhood. If lifestyle when developed, prevented from smoking, overeating, bad habits. If children adopt good habits of eating, exercise and not forming bad habits, these diseases can be prevented. It is done through individual and mass education.

Primary Prevention

Action taken prior to the onset of disease that removes possibility that disease will ever occur. Promoting general health and well-being, quality of life and specific protection. Maintaining an acceptable level of health that will enable every individual to lead a socially, economically productive life. Strategy for this is, population strategy and high-risk strategy. Behavioral and lifestyle changes and risk group identification.

Secondary Prevention

Action which halts the progress of disease and prevents complications. Early diagnosis by screening tests, case finding program and adequate treatment.

Tertiary Prevention

When disease process has advanced beyond its early stages then tertiary prevention is done. All measures available to reduce or limit impairment and disabilities and minimize suffering caused by existing condition and promote patient's adjustment to irremediable condition.

Modes of intervention are health promotion, specific protection, early diagnosis and treatment, disability limitation and rehabilitation. Health promotion is by health education, environmental modification, nutritional interventions, lifestyle and behavioral changes.

Health services are usually organized at three levels:

1. Primary health care
2. Secondary health care
3. Tertiary health care.

Primary Health Care

This is the first level of contact between individual and the health system where essential health care, primary health care is provided. Majority of health problems can be dealt with, at this level. In Indian context, this care is provided by the primary health centers and their subcenters with community participation.

Secondary Health Care

At this level, more complex problems are dealt with. This care comprises of essentially curative services and is provided by the district hospitals and community health centers or rural hospitals. This level serves as first referral level in health system.

Tertiary Health Care

This level offers superspecialist care. This care is provided by the regional central level institutions. These institutions provide not only highly specialized care, but also planning and managerial skills and teaching for specialized staff. This level supports actions carried out at primary level.

MODERN CONCEPT OF HEALTHCARE APPROACH

Primary Healthcare Approach

It is a new approach to health care that initiates at the community level; all the factors required for improving health status of population. It consists of at least eight elements described as essential health care. Simple and efficient health care with regard to cost, technology and organization that are readily accessible to those concerned and that contributes to improve the living conditions of individuals, families and community as a whole. It is available to all people at the first level of health care. Principles are wider coverage, equity, individual and community involvement, and intersectoral coordination.

Risk Approach or Risk Group Approach

It consists of identifying the risk groups or target groups. For example, at risk mothers, at risk infants, at risk families, chronically ill, handicapped, elderly, sexually transmitted infection (STI) cases. Risk approach is something for all, but more for those in need in proportion to the need.

Regulatory Approach

Regulatory or legal approach seeks to protect the health of public through the enforcement of law and regulations. For example, Epidemic Disease Act, Food Adulteration Act.

Service Approach

Providing all the health facilities needed by the community.

Educational Approach

Educational approach is major means today for achieving change in health practices and the recognition of health. Promoting general health and well-being, quality of life and specific protection. Maintaining an acceptable level of health that will enable every individual to lead a socially and economically productive life. Strategy for this is population strategy and high-risk strategy. Behavioral and lifestyle changes and risk group identification.

ROLE OF NURSE IN GIVING PRIMARY HEALTH CARE

Multipurpose health workers, female and male are basic health workers giving primary health care. Health assistants, female and male are supervisors of these workers.

There is subcenter for every 5,000 population and in hilly areas for 3,000 population. They will function as member of health team and provide basic health care.

- Family health care—survey, identify high-risk mothers and infants, cases of communicable diseases

- Environmental sanitation, safe water, immunizations
- Emergency medicines in communicable diseases
- Reproductive and child health care—antenatal, intranatal, postnatal and under 5 care
- Supervise anganwadi workers regarding growth and development, assessment of children, diet, nutritional supplements to children, antenatal care (ANC) and postnatal care (PNC) cases
- Motivate couples for family planning and adopting various methods for it
- Follow-up of all cases
- Prepare slides of blood and sputum for malaria and tuberculosis indentification and send to laboratory for confirmation of diagnosis
- Give treatment of malaria and tuberculosis as per order (DOT)
- Educate people regarding personal hygiene, environmental sanitation, diet, habits, prevention of communicable diseases, family welfare, immunizations, MTP, copper T, and operation of tubectomy and vasectomy.

CHAPTER

2

Nursing as a Profession

AIM

Students understand what is nursing, nursing as a profession, ethics and responsibility.

OBJECTIVES

- Students know what is nursing
- Students understand the concept of professional nursing
- Students know the ethical principles in nursing practice
- Students know the various roles a nurse performs.

PROFESSION

Definition

Profession is defined as an occupation with ethical components that is devoted to the promotion of human and social welfare.
According to Abraham Flexner, Profession has essential intellectual operations, large individual responsibility learnt in nature, techniques of communication through highly specialized educational discipline, self-organized activities and responsibilities.

Characteristics

Advanced body of knowledge and skills, code of ethics or organized value system, academic preparation, professional socialization, intellectual operations, well-organized structure to assume required level of education and practice, undivided responsibility, vital service to humanity, devotion to responsibilities and patient care, meeting social needs.

NURSING

Definition

International Council of Nurses (ICN) has accepted definition of nursing by **Virginia Henderson** "The unique function of nurse is to assist the individual, sick or well, in the performance of those activities contributing to health or its recovery, or to peaceful death that he would perform unaided if he had the necessary strength, will or knowledge and to do this in such a way as to help him to gain independence as rapidly as possible". Nurse is a person who has completed a program of basic nursing education and is qualified and authorized to her country to supply the most responsible services of a nursing nature for promotion of health, prevention of illness and care of the sick.

American Nursing Association (ANA) 2003: Nursing is the protection, promotion and optimization of health and abilities, prevention of illness and injury, alleviation of suffering through the diagnosis and treatment of human responses and advocacy in the care of individuals, families, communities and population.

Faye Abdellah emphasizes delivering nursing care for the whole person, to meet the physical, emotional, intellectual, social and spiritual needs of the client and family.

According to Florence Nightingale: A nurse must be no gossip, no vain talker. She should never answer questions about her sick, except to those who have right to ask about them. She must be a religious and devoted woman, she must have respect for own calling, because God's precious gift of life is often so literally placed in her hands. She must be sound, close and quick observer, she must be a woman of delicate and decent feelings.

Philosophy

Nurses believe that nursing contributes to health services to meet the health goals and nurses participate in healthcare programs. Nursing practice includes hospital-based curative and rehabilitative practices and preventive, promotive activities for health. Nurses care for patients and help them to be independent in self-care. They use knowledge base, standard nursing practice skills and attitude of caring and empathy in patient care. Nurses apply many theories of nursing in practice, identify patient's health needs, plan and implement the care and evaluate. They use knowledge base for clinical judgment, standard skills for practice and work with responsibility. They follow code of ethics and protect patient's rights and human rights.

Objectives

- A graduate nurse is able to identify patient's health needs, plan a care, implement and evaluate
- Uses knowledge base, critical thinking and make the clinical judgments
- Able to use various healthcare techniques and machines, instruments in caring
- Participates as a member of health team effectively
- Demonstrates leadership and managerial skills in the clinical and community settings
- Demonstrates professional attitude, self-development, quality care, good citizenship and teamwork
- To establish and promote implementation of standards of nursing practice, nursing education and nursing service as defined by statutory bodies
- To encourage the members to adhere to the ethical obligations of nurses as patient advocates
- To promote and protect economic and general welfare of the nurses.

NATURE AND SCOPE OF NURSING PRACTICE

A profession is one, which utilizes in its practice a well-defined and well-organized body of specialized knowledge, which is on the intellectual level of the higher learning. It constantly enlarges body of knowledge and uses and improves techniques of education and service by use of scientific method. It entrusts the education of the practitioners to institutions for higher education. It applies body of knowledge in the practical services, which are vital to human and social welfare. It functions autonomously in the formation of professional policy and in the control of professional activity. It attracts individuals of intellectual and personal qualities who exalt services above personal gain and who recognize their chosen occupation as a lifework. It strives to compensate its practitioners by providing freedom of action, opportunity for continuous professional growth and economic security.

FUNCTIONS OF A NURSE

As a Caregiver

A nurse helps the patient to regain health through the healing process. It is not just the cure of a disease and treatment skills, but includes measures to restore emotional, spiritual and social well-being. She helps the patient and family to set goals and meet them with minimum cost, time and energy.

As an Advocate

She protects patient's human and legal rights and assists them. Assistance may be in communication and decision-making conflicts.

As an Educator

She helps for the promotion of health, self-care and demonstrates certain procedures. As a communicator, she is resource person for the patient, family and health personnel. She assists with rehabilitation and continuation of care.

As a Manager

She coordinates all activities concerned with the patient to the members of the health team. She uses critical thinking skills for effective care. Nurses provide direct client care in many settings, in hospital using nursing process. Restorative and curative care is provided. Advance practice nurse functions independently in many countries. Clinical nurse specialist is expert in specialized area of practice. Nurse practitioner provides healthcare to clients in ambulatory setting, outpatient departments and in the community. Acute care nurse works in acute care setting in hospital or special clinics. Geriatric nurse cares for older adults. Certified nurse midwife is a registered nurse and provides independent care to mothers during pregnancy, childbirth and postnatal care. Pediatric nurse is specialized for care of children. Psychiatric nurse and public health nurse work in psychiatric field and community respectively. Nurse educators work in nursing schools and colleges. Neonatal nurses work in neonatal setting. Oncological nurses work in cancer care units. Auxiliary nursing personnel work in maternity wards, private clinics, and rural areas of community.

Responsibilities of Registered Nurse Midwife

Fundamental responsibility of a registered or enlisted nurse is to conserve life, alleviate sufferings and promote health. She/he maintains, at all time, the highest standard of nursing care and professional conduct and shall not be only prepared to practice, but also shall maintain her knowledge and skill at constantly high-level. She/he shall not only recognize the responsibility, but also the limitations of the professional functions. Shall give medical treatment without medical order, only in emergency and report such actions to physician at the earliest possible moment. She/he shall carry out physician's orders intelligently and with loyalty, but shall refuse to participate in unethical procedures and notify the proper authorities if any, such conduct of her associates. She/he shall sustain confidence in the physician and other members of the health team and cooperate and maintain harmonious relationship. She/he shall adhere to the standards of personal ethics which will reflect upon the profession.

QUALITIES OF A NURSE

Physically healthy, intelligent, thoughtful, emotionally stable, well-mannered, considerate, technically competent, alert, with ability to observe and interpret, able to communicate effectively, dependable and trustworthy, sensitive, confident, resourceful, open-minded, courageous, punctual, responsible and sincere.

CATEGORIES OF NURSING PERSONNEL

Nurses work in various settings according to their qualification.

- Nursing service
- Nursing education
- Nursing research.

Registered nurse, registered midwife, registered nurse-midwife, graduate nurse, postgraduates, nurse administrators, nurse educator, departmental supervisor, departmental sister, ward incharge sister, pediatric nurse, psychiatric nurse, theater nurse, ICU nurse, renal specialist nurses, community health nurses, auxiliary nurse midwife, health assistants, multipurpose health worker female/male, oncological nurses.

HISTORY OF NURSING

Knowledge of history of nursing will help us to know how nursing began, who contributed towards its development, and how nursing profession developed in the past three centuries. We will be able to compare the nursing in the past and present and will be able to understand the changes in future, roles and responsibilities.

Year 5000 BC—Ayurvedic medicine started. Dhanwantari, the physician of God is believed to appear during Samudramanthanam.

Year 4000 BC—In Greece, Unani and Homeopathy were practiced.

Year 2100 BC—King Samurai, a Babilonion emperor developed a code of law for the doctors and nurses. Medicines were herbal and very bitter. Team approach was used.

Year 2000 BC—In China, medicine and surgery were honored callings. They were allowed to practice dissection and described internal organs. They knew about circulation of blood. Sen Lung was known as the Father of Medicine in China. He used many vegetables and animals in medicine. There was a belief that touching a sick person might give entry to evil spirit. In Hans Dynasty, the first woman attending sick was Chun Yu Yan, the first midwife.

Year 1600 BC—In Greece, superstitions and magic were practiced. Records were written on papyrus paper. It contained records of disease, drugs, and surgery. Imhotep, a priest physician, was liked by everyone due to his kind personality. Women had some freedom. Mother had position of authority. They nursed sick at home.

Year 1400 BC—In India, Sushruta known as the Father of Surgery, wrote a book on surgery. Charaka, a physician, wrote Charaka Samhita, a book on internal medicine. Charaka was raj vaidya to king Kanishka. Sarpagandha, a medicine for hypertension, is still used. Hospitals were large and well-equipped.

Year 1200 BC—In Greece, Aesculapius was the king. His two daughters, Hygeia and Panacea, were called as goddess of health and medicine. It was believed that medicine is of divine origin and represented by many Gods. Apollo, the Sun, was God of health and medicine. Aesculapius son was God of healing. Temples were built for these Gods and the priest physicians were in charge. Sick people came for treatment and cure. Treatment included diet, massage, bath and inunction.

Year 1000 BC—Physiotherapy was practiced in China. They knew vaccination. Romans and Greeks migrated to Ireland and regulated practice of medicine.

Year 800 BC—In ancient India, renowned authorities in Ayurveda were Sushruta, Charaka, Vagbhata and Atreya.

Year 550 BC—Cyrus the great, became leader of Medes and Persians. They believed in evil spirit theory of disease and practiced spiritual assistance in cure.

Year 460 BC—Hippocrates, son of a priest physician, known as the Father of Medicine taught that evil spirit did not cause disease, but that is due to man's disobedience of the laws of nature. It was the beginning of scientific medicine. He taught to observe signs and symptoms and come to diagnosis. He developed ways of physical examination and taking history. He stressed fresh air, cleanliness and good diet for health. Caduceus insignia for medicine is a symbol associated with Aesculapius.

Year 272–236 BC—King Ashoka built monasteries, houses for travelers, hospitals for men and animals in India. Prevention of disease and hygienic practice was adopted. Doctors and midwives were to be trustworthy and skillful. They had to wear clean clothes and keep their nails short. Rooms were kept clean and well-ventilated. Nurses were usually men and old women.

Year 1–500 AD—Early Christian era, superstitions and magic were replaced by update practice. Nursing was nurtured in this period. There were three groups of Christian women known as apostolic orders. They were either unmarried or widows who devoted themselves to the service of other women. They had status of Decon, a servant. Deacons and Deaconesses were visiting the houses of the poor and sick. They provided food and money and prayed for them. They gave medicines according to their knowledge and ability. Phoebe was a Greek lady, deaconess from south Italy who helped the sick at their houses. She was honored as world's first deaconess and first visiting nurse and forerunner of modern public health nurse. Among three orders of women, first order was the Deaconesses who were mature women assisted by clergy went out teaching, preaching and caring for the sick. Second order was of widows assisted with house visiting. Third order was virgins who were younger women who cared for church vestment and gave out arms to poor. There was another group of women known as Roman matrons. In Rome, women of high rank had much freedom. They were interested in charity and nursing. They founded monastries and hospitals. Marcella, very rich and educated lady, turned her palace into monastery and did charitable work. Fabiola was a young beautiful lady from persian family, became Christian under the influence of Marcella and turned her home to free Christian hospital in 390 AD. Paula was a friend of Fabiola. She made hospice for travelers and hospital for the sick. She and her daughter Eustachium and other women did nursing. Deaconesses opened their homes for the poor and became known as Diaconia. As these houses were not sufficient, more rooms were added called as Xenodochium and they took care of the strangers, sick, insanes, lapers, orphans, aged and travelers. St Basil built a hospital at Caesarea in Palestine. Macarena was in charge of the hospital. Deaconesses served as nurses. Helena, Mother of emperor Constantine, helped to build many hospitals and churches in Rome. In North America, there were several groups of people as Mayas, Incas and Aztecs. They used sweatbath as medicinal remedy. They practiced human sacrifices to cure illness. They removed hearts from young adults and children. In the time of stress, maidens were thrown in sacred well. Inca in Peru were treating diseases with bloodletting, cupping, massaging, sweating, splinting, setting bones, tooth extraction, amputation, suturing, bandaging, poulticing and trephining. Art of medicine, nursing and pharmacy were combined first in medicine man and later in priest physician. In medicine, two outstanding professionals were Celsus and Galen. Celsus was a Roman patrician in the first century. He had his education in Alexandra and Egypt. He was known as the Founder of Experimental Physiology and popular teacher of anatomy. He wrote eight books on amputation, plastic surgery, hernias, venesection, cataract and other operations. These became chief Arab medical resources. St Luke, Greek Evangelist, a doctor was called as a beloved physician. St Cosmas and St Damian Arab, twin brothers were specialized in medicine and pharmacy and practiced medicine in Asia minor. Soranus of Ephesus, Greek obstetrician and pediatrician was a student of great school of Alexandra. He wrote many practical medical books and studied muscles, glands and nerves.

Year 500–1500 AD—Middle ages. In the history of the world, the period is divided into ancient, medieval, and modern history. Middle ages are medieval period. After the attack of barbaric tribes, Rome was disorganized. Roman armies were dismissed, roads and bridges were destroyed. Homes were destroyed. Romans moved to Constantinople. People who were not able to move, approached monasteries for help and protection. Monte Casino was built between Rome and Naples. St Benedict of Persia encouraged all to become Christian and work together. These monasteries became chief place for education, medicine and nursing. Women were given freedom to develop their own skills and ideas. Men and women had separate monasteries and had to use distinctive dress. The veils, part of convent dress symbolized humanity, obedience and service. The cap of modern nurse is a modification of the religious veil and associated with humanity and rendering services to mankind. St Brigit introduced female monasteries in Ireland. She was scholar, counselor and healer. She cared for the sick. She was labeled as patroness of healing. St Scolastic twin sister of St Benedict, founded Benedictine community for women. This order was established near Monte Casino and she became its abbess, a female superior. Abbots and abbesses were heads of monasteries with fiefs, a piece of land given by king. Serfs were to fight at the time of war and treated as slaves. They had to cultivate and give the yield to Baron. To remove quarrels amongst steers and Barons and knights, church gave training to knights. This was known as Chivalry. Three hospitals were built in France, Hotel Dieu of Lyons, Hotel Dieu of Paris and the Santo Spirito Hospital, Rome. Hotel Dieu of Lyons was built by king Chilbert. Management was by lay persons and workers were penitents and widows. Later on, Augustinian sisters managed the nursing and routine work of washing, feeding and giving medicine. Again in 16th century, men called rectors managed it. Hospital had large beds to accommodate five patients. Rectors thought of providing separate bed for each patient. Then hospital had 1100 beds. Nurses were from pleasant class between 16–24 years of age. Each nurse was assigned 15–20 patients for the day and 100 for nights. Wards were large—32 feet wide and 25 feet high and separate ward for different disease. Nurses had no training. Once they became nun, they had to be for life. They had to work without servants. Hotel Dieu of Paris lay women organized themselves in religious body and adopted the rule of St Augustine and became Augustinian sisters. Brothers in male wards and sisters for female wards. They cared for patients and took charge of kitchen and laundry. King of Western Saxon built Santo Spirito hospital in Rome. It had 1,000 beds. These three hospitals are still existing. Three military nursing orders, were formed to undertake healthcare services, (1) Order of Knights, hospital of St John, (2) Teutonic Knights in Germany and (3) Order of Knights of St Lazarus. Two hostels were built for warfare relief work. Men working were dedicated to St John. Hospitallers was formed. They were divided into three classes—warriors, nurses and spiritual. Knights of St Lazarus gave specialized care for leprosy patients. St Hildegirde, St Elizabeth of Hungary cared for patients. St Catherine of Siena hospital cared for lepers. She cared for patients day and night in La Scala hospital.

Year 1664 AD—Building was set apart for soldiers in Chennai. This was forerunner of general hospital, Chennai.

Year 1707—First hospital was opened in Kolkata by the council of Fort William for soldiers.

Year 1753—Twelve houses with gardens were acquired for St George's hospital, Chennai.

Year 1768—In Kolkata, Kirnander's house was bought and converted to hospital, now known as Seth Sukhlal Karnani Memorial Hospital. Matron was Ms Abraham, who came to Kolkata in 1928 bringing qualified nurses with her.

Year 1784—In Mumbai, a hospital was opened in fort for Europeans and another on Esplanade for sepoy and third for convalescent on adjacent island.

Year 1809—Hospital for Indians was opened in Bombay with 20 beds and Indian dispensary.

Year 1820—Florence Nightingale was born on 12th may in Italy.

Year 1832—Catholic order, the sisters of charity started by Catherine, M Auley in Ireland, started nursing in Dublin hospital and then went all over the world.

Year 1838—Kolkata Medical College and Hospital was started with 30 beds and OPD. At Neyyoor, London Mission Hospital was opened.

Year 1840—Elizabeth Fry, with her sister and daughter, organized Protestant Sisters of Charity. They went to work in Guy's hospital for a few hours a day under the supervision of doctors and untrained ward sisters. They became nursing attendants in private homes. Amelia Sieveking started home visiting association in Hamburg, Germany. Nurses had poor manners, lack of education, bad habits as written in book by Charles Dickens made public aware of the need for reform. Dorothea Lynde Dix was called the John Howard of America for work of caring for mentally ill and criminals. She formed a basis of present system of mental hospitals. She worked in England and Europe.

Year 1843—J J Hospital was founded at the joint expenses of East India Company and Sir Jamshedjee Jeejeebhoy in Bombay.

Year 1849—Florence Nightingale visited Europe and observed convent nuns, their mode of life. She met Mr and Mrs Sydney Herbert and heard their plan to start a hospital in England.

Year 1850—St John house was established by church of England to give systematic training to nurses in hospital. Nurses from both the orders went to Crimea with Florence Nightingale.

Year 1852—Florence visited Alexandria, Egypt, and observed work of Sisters of Charity of St Vincent D Paul. She studied at American school and orphanage. She visited many hospitals in Germany. She visited Kaiserworth hospital for two weeks and joined for three months training. At the age of 33, she became superintendent of an establishment for gentle women during sickness. In Crimean war, Russia and France had religious sisters to care for their soldiers. England had only untrained men. Sidney Herbert asked her to take responsibility to take band of nurses to Crimea. With 38 nurses selected from catholic and protestant orders from the hospital went to Crimea. At Scutari, there were two hospitals. She was given Barrack hospital with 1500 patients. Wards were crowded, dirty, poorly ventilated. Patients were on floor. No basins, soap, towels or clothing available. She proved her ability in adverse conditions and in emergencies, she used her own money. She maintained cleanliness, bathed patients, provided clean linen. In 6 months of time, hospital was reformed. She spent her evening visiting the sick and writing letters for soldiers.

Year 1856—Peace was declared and hospitals were closed. Her work at war was appreciated and people wanted to honor her. Nightingale fund was raised for nursing training schools. She wrote books—notes on hospital, notes on nursing.

Year 1860—Nightingale School was opened in June with 15 students. Nightingale graduates were sent to establish nursing schools in England, America and all parts of the world. Miss Linda Richards was the first American trained nurse. Lady Hardinge hospital, Shimla, Civil Hospital, Amritsar started nursing school. Hospital was built and Miss MF MacDonnell was nursing superintendent. Jackman Memorial Hospital was started at Bilaspur, Indore, Ratlam, and Friend's Mission Hospital at Hoshangabad, Madhya Pradesh. There were training schools for nursing under United Church of Canada Mission. Cowasji Jehangir Ophthalmic Hospital was opened in J J Hospital Mumbai. David and Jacob Sassoon Hospitals were founded in Pune. St Stephen Hospital was established in Delhi.

Year 1867—Government General Hospital Chennai, established a plan to train nurses and six nurses were trained who were from England.

Year 1871—Bellevue hospital training school started in New York.

Year 1873—GT Hospital, Mumbai, was founded. Mayo Indian Hospital was opened in Kolkata.

Year 1874—Nursing school was opened in Sassoon Hospital, Pune.

Year 1877—Sisters community of all saints came to India from England. Cama and Albless Hospital was established in Mumbai. Sister Eleanor Mary was nursing superintendent of J J Hospital Mumbai.

Year 1884—Government of Bombay asked sisters of all saint community to take responsibility of nursing in Fort George Hospital, now St George Hospital.

Year 1885—Victoria caste Hospital started in Egmore.

Year 1886—Miss Atkinson, a Nightingale nurse, joined Cama Hospital Mumbai.

Year 1887—Miss Bedford Fenwick formed association of trained nurses. Nursing sisters were sent out by the government to organize nursing in military hospitals. Indian Army Nursing service was laid down. First nursing superintendent was Miss Locke, who was trained in Bartholomew's Hospital, London, and her assistant was Ms Foxley. Miss Locke with five sisters stationed at Rawalpindi, now in Pakistan, and miss Foxley with three sisters in Bengaluru.

Year 1888—St George's Hospital, Mumbai was founded. Shatani Dhankorabai opened Canada Hospital, Nashik.

Year 1891—First Indian lady to join nursing in J J Hospital, Smt Kashibai Ganpati, sent from Thane municipality. St Columbia Hospital Hazaribagh, Sir William, Wanless Hospital, Miraj started.

Year 1892—Kugler Hospital, Guntur, started. Bowring and Lady Carson Hospital started in Bengaluru.

Year 1895—Mrs Vsterman and Miss Hope looked after training nurses and reached very high standard in Bowring Hospital. St Margaret Hospital Pune, started. Nursing school started at Wanless Hospital, Miraj.

Year 1897—Shambhu Nath Hospital opened in Kolkata and training of nurses started. Christian Medical College and Hospital, Vellore, was started by Dr Ida Scudder. Miss Delia Houghton, American nurse, came for nursing in CMC, Vellore.

Year 1901—Public health nursing with child welfare work started in Finland. Infant welfare center started in Paris.

Year 1907–09—Sevasadan Society formed by wife of justice Ranade, sent many widows for nursing training at Sassoon Hospital, Pune. These nurses later on, supervised nurses at Solapur. Sayaji Hospital in Gujarat was also conducting nursing training. Conference of nursing and medical superintendents was organized and North India United Board of Examiners for Mission Hospitals was formed. Bombay Presidency Nursing Association was formed, which laid down curriculum for nursing schools and also started inspections and maintained registration of trained nurses. Lady Hardinge Hospital in Delhi started.

Year 1911—King George's Hospital in Lucknow started medical college and nursing school.

Year 1913–14—Nurses were recruited in India being attached to Queen Alexandra's Military and Indian Station Hospitals.

Year 1915—Lady Hardinge Medical College started in Delhi. Sister Gregory was founder member of North Indian Board of Mission. Dutches Hospital started in Patna, Bihar.

Year 1916—KEM Hospital, Mumbai, started and nursing school was opened.

Year 1923—Mrs Holden established well-organized training school in Mure Memorial Hospital, Nagpur, and Miss S Steem was Nursing Superintendent. School of Nursing in Clough Memorial Hospital, Ongole, started by Miss Sigrid Johnson, Mission hospitals were started at Khammam, Medak, Hanamkonda and Shillong. Miss Bullock was Matron in Welsh Hospital and she was also the first superintendent of nursing services in Assam. Mahatma Gandhi Hospital, Jodhpur and Jaipur, Zanana Hospital were founded. Osmania Hospital, Hyderabad, was started.

Year 1926—Indian Military nursing service started with 12 matrons, 18 sisters, and 25 staff nurses. Nursing training school started at Visakhapatnam, Chennai and Guwahti.

Year 1929—Bai Jerbai Wadia Hospital, Mumbai, started and opened a nursing school matron being Lorna Mackenzie st George's Hospital trainee.

Year 1935—Nursing training started in GT Hospital Mumbai, and in Irwin Hospital, New Delhi.

Year 1937—Central Advisory Board of Health was formed.

Year 1939—Safdarjung Hospital started as military hospital in Delhi. Holy Family Hospital, Patna, started.

Year 1942—Safdarjung Hospital was handed over to Government as a general hospital. Auxiliary nursing service started due to shortage of nursing staff. About 3,000 women in India were given 6 months training and enrolled in the auxiliary nursing service. Miss EE Hutchinson became the Chief Nursing Superintendent of ANS and an Advisor to Government of India. Four years BSc Nursing program was started in Rajkumari Amrit Kaur College of Nursing and Christian Medical College and Hospital, Vellore.

Year 1946—Miss Florence Tailor, MSc Nursing, joined as dean College of nursing, CMC Vellore.

Year 1948—Miss Adrenwala became the first Trained Nurses Association of India (TNAI) President. She also became the first Secretary of Indian Nursing Council, when it was constituted. Manipur Hospital started with Mrs A Thomas as the matron.

Year 1950—School of Nursing was started at Dhamtari Christian Hospital, MPSr Lena Graber as matron with four students. In CMC Vellore, Miss Anna Jacob, Indian nurse, took charge as the Nursing Superintendent.

Year 1951—Two years ANM training was started at Tarn Taran, Punjab, in St Mary Hospital.

Year 1953—First Post Certificate Public Health Nursing course started at All India Institute of Public Health, Kolkata. The United Nations Children's Fund (UNICEF) was formed.

Year 1955—First nursing audit.

Year 1956—Miss Adrenwala received Florence Nightingale Medal and became Nursing Advisor to Government of India.

Year 1957—Miss Buchanan became Principal of RAK College of nursing.

Year 1958—Lady Reading School, Delhi, started. BSc Nursing started at SNDT University.

Year 1960—First MSc Nursing batch started at RAK College of Nursing, Delhi.

Year 1962—Four Years BSc Nursing course started at J J Hospital, Mumbai.

Year 1963—263 ANM Schools were started in India.

Year 1966—First two years PC BSc Nursing course started at Thiruvananthapuram.

Year 1968—Two years and six months duration of PC BSc Nursing and MSc Nursing was started at CMC Vellore.

Year 1972—Two years PC BSc Nursing course was started at Institute of Nursing Education, JJ Hospital, Mumbai.

Year 1977—ANM course revised by Indian Nursing Council and named as multipurpose health worker course of 18 months. Preventive aspects like genetic counseling, coronary heart disease and cancer were added to National Health programs.

Year 1980—Screening serological tests, high-risk group identification, health check-up and population policy was included in public health programs.

Year 1981—Health for all by 2000 AD Alma Ata Declaration. Primary health care started.

Year 1982—GNM syllabus was revised by Indian Nursing Council (INC) and duration was made three years.

Year 1983—Four years BSc Nursing course started at Choithram College of Nursing in Indore.

Year 1985—In America, hospitals are reimbursed at fix rate and, therefore, hospital stay was shortened. Home health care became alternative. Home care nursing interventions include IV therapy, injections, venipuncture, catheterization, pressure ulcer treatments, wound care, ostomy care and health education.

Year 1988—Miss Pauline E King received, national best nurse award.

Year 1989—First batch of oncological nursing started at Tata Memorial Hospital, Mumbai.

Year 1995—Cairo Conference. Holistic approach in the Royal children's Hospital (RCH) was introduced.

Year 1996—Target free approach in family welfare program. First batch of BSc Nursing graduates was out in College of Nursing, Bharati Vidyapeeth, Pune. MSc Nursing started in Bengaluru.

Year 1998—Maharashtra University of Health Sciences came into existence at Nashik.

Year 2000—Miss Adrenwala passed away in Ruby Health Clinic, Pune.

Year 2001—MSc Nursing started at Bharati Vidyapeeth, Pune.

Year 2003—Five new nursing colleges were opened at Wardha, Pune, Navi Mumbai, Jalgaon.

NURSING AS A PROFESSION

Essential components of nursing care are—care, cure and coordination.

Care

Providing comfort and support in the time of anxiety, loneliness and helplessness. It is listening, evaluating and intervening appropriately.

Cure

Promotion of health and healing. Assisting patients to understand their health problems and helping them to cope. Administering medicine and treatment. Using clinical judgment, on the basis of patient's reactions and plan a care. How to use existing and potential resources to help the patient towards recovery and adjustment by mobilizing their own resources.

Coordination

It is coordinating medical and other professional and technical services for the patients. It is supervising, teaching and directing all those who give nursing care.

VALUES

Values are beliefs or attitudes about the worth of a person, object, idea or action. Value systems are basic to way of life and give direction to life, form basis of behavior, especially on decisions or choices. Values are personal and professional. Professional values are code of ethics.

Values in Professional Nursing

Strong commitment to service, belief and dignity and worth of each person, commitment to education and professional autonomy.
Altruism: Concern for well-being of others.
Autonomy: Right to self-determination.
Human dignity: Respect individual.
Integrity: Working with accepted standards of practice and code of Ethics.
Social justice: Upholding of moral, legal and humanistic principles.

Caring

Caring promotes common good or welfare of group. Caring is central force in client-nurse relationship, force for protecting and enhancing client's dignity. Carrying out nursing activities with compassion, with empathetic understanding, and with respect for the patient as individual of worth and dignity in caring. Part of caring function is providing comfort, support to patient and family, helping to regain his independence. Helping him to meet his daily needs of water, food, rest, sleep and maintain normal body functioning.

Advocacy

Protect client's rights. Right to safety, right to be informed, right to choose, right to be heard, right to seek redressal, and right to consumer education.

ETHICS

Definition

Ethics is a formal, systematic study of moral beliefs. Ethics are the rules or principles that govern the right conduct.
Utilitarian Theory: " The greatest of good for greatest number"
Deontological or Formalist Theory: Moral standards or principles exist independently of the ends or consequences. The word Ethics is derived from Greek word 'Ethos', means custom or guiding belief. Ethics are characteristics of a profession and are called as "code". Ethics deal with what is good and bad with moral duty and obligations.

Ethics is a study of good conduct, character and motives. Ethics is code of moral principles. Nursing ethics is the code governing a nurse's behavior with patients and relatives and with colleagues.

Ethical Principles

Autonomy

Self-rule, ability to make choice, free from external constraints. Nurse should be able to work confidently and independently. She has to identify patients health needs on her own, plan, implement and evaluate the care.

Beneficence

The duty to do well. Promoting goodness, kindness and charity.

Confidentiality

Privacy; information obtained from the patient will not be disclosed to another unless it will benefit the person or there is direct threat to social good.

Fidelity

Promise keeping. To be faithful to one's commitment.

Justice

Clients should be treated alike. Each person receives services equally, according to need, according to efforts, legal entitlement, irrespective of caste, creed, religion and race.

Respect for Persons

All should be respected.

Veracity

Obligation to tell the truth and not to lie or deceive others.

Nonmaleficence

Avoidance of harm or hurt. Ethical practice involves not only the will to do good, but also equal commitment to do no harm.

Code of Ethics by International Council of Nurses

Nursing ethics is concerned with the moral obligations, which regulate the nurse's performance of her duties. The following code of ethics is based on the recommendations made by the International Council of Nurses, Frankfurt, Germany 1965. A Nurse has three fundamental responsibilities—to conserve life, to alleviate sufferings and to promote health. The nurse shall maintain at all times the highest standards of nursing care and of professional conduct. The nurse must not only be prepared for practice, but shall maintain knowledge and skill at a constantly high-level. The religious beliefs of a patient shall be respected. Nurses hold in confidence all the personal information entrusted to them. Nurses recognize not only the responsibilities but also the limitations for their professional functions. They do not recommend or give medical treatment without medical orders, except in emergencies and they report such actions to a physician as soon as possible. The nurse is under obligation to carry out the physician's orders intelligently and to refuse to participate in unethical procedures. The nurse sustains confidence in the physician and other members of the health team. Incompetence or unethical conduct of associate should be exposed but only to proper authority. The nurse is entitled to just remuneration and accepts only such compensation as the contract, actual or implied, provides. Nurses do not permit their names to be used in connection with the advertisement of products or with any other forms of self-advertisement. The nurse cooperates and maintains harmonious relationship with the members of other profession and with the nursing colleagues. The nurse adheres to the standards of personal ethics, which reflect credit upon the profession. In personal conduct, nurses should not knowingly disregard the accepted pattern of behavior of the community, in which they live and work. The nurse participates and shares responsibility with other citizens and other health professionals in promoting efforts to meet health needs of public—local, state, national and international.

NURSE'S PLEDGE

"I solemnly pledge myself before God and in the presence of this assembly to pass my life in purity and to practice my profession faithfully. I will abstain from whatever is deleterious and mischievous and will not take or knowingly administer any harmful drug. I will do all in my power to maintain and elevate the standard of my profession and will hold in confidence all personal matters committed to my keeping and all family affairs coming to my knowledge in the practice of my profession. With loyalty, I will endeavor to aid the physician in his work and devote myself to the welfare of those committed to my care".

CHAPTER 3

Patient's Admission to Hospital, Discharge and Transfer

AIM

Students are able to admit the patient and follow the protocol of transfer and discharge.

OBJECTIVES

- Students know the admission procedure
- Students know the discharge procedure and the responsibility of nurse in educating patient regarding follow-up and health check-up, health habits
- Students know how to transfer a patient from one ward to another and to other hospital.

ADMISSION TO HOSPITAL

Clients may be admitted to hospital for investigations, health check-up, disease condition, surgery, childbirth, accidents and emergencies. Admission will depend on the condition of the patient, stage of the disease, treatment required, age and sex of the patient and type of assistance needed.

They may be admitted to emergency ward, intensive care unit (ICU), neonatal intensive care unit (NICU), pediatric ward, gynecology ward, labor ward, surgical or medical ward, isolation ward, plastic surgery ward, orthopedic ward, burns ward, neurosurgery ward. Usually, clients are examined in outpatient department, casualty and according to need they are hospitalized.

It may be routine admission or emergency admission. Emergency admission requires admission bed, resuscitation equipment, emergency drugs, oxygen, suctioning equipment, portable X-ray machine, stretcher, IV fluids and are kept ready in emergency ward and casualty. Client is transferred to related ward when he or she is in a condition to transfer. Medicolegal cases observation is made and recorded. Clothes, gastric fluid, blood samples, etc. are preserved. When blood transfusion is needed, grouping and cross matching is done and blood is arranged immediately. Patient may need emergency surgery and prepared for operation immediately.

Psychological Aspect of Illness and Patient's Reaction to Admission

- Sudden change or strangeness in the environment produces fear and anxiety
- Entering the hospital is a threat to one's personal identity
- Admission to hospital creates stress on physical and psychological health
- People have different lifestyles, habits, modes of behavior, which are affected by admission to hospital
- Absence from job and responsibilities at home creates tension
- Patients with medicolegal procedures may find it difficult to stay and have behavior problems
- Fear of operation, death, sights of other serious patients increases fear and tension
- Restriction of visitors, hindered communication may create helplessness
- Procedures like injection, intravenous infusions, tube feeding, enema creates fear, especially in children
- Children are afraid of doctors, nurses in uniforms, instruments and too many people present in ward
- Restriction on diet, activities, behavior creates tension
- Economic problems, if present may trouble a patient when paying bills, purchase of drugs, articles and staying someone nextkin and their food
- Needs which are physiological, psychological, social and spiritual, if met, patient adjusts to environment of the hospital.

Unit and Its Preparation

Room temperature: 18–24°C.
Humidity: 60–70%, curtains for windows.
Type of bed: As required—simple, Fowler's, cardiac, orthopedic, railings.
Mattress: Cotton, coir, water, air.
Overhead table. Pillow under head, extra pillows for comfort.
Backrest, bolster, footboard, stockings, splints as required.
Mackintosh, bed linen, screen, mouthwash tray, saline stand, thermometer, sphygmomanometer, central nervous system (CNS) tray, kidney tray or emesis basin, urinal, bedpan, bucket, mug, jug with drinking water, glass or feeding cup.
Personal belongings—toothbrush, paste, comb, soap in soapdish, towels, hand washing articles, gown, mask, gloves, if communicable disease present.

Make admission bed, keep bed warm, keep charts and book ready.

Admission Procedure

Patients are admitted routinely for deficiency diseases, chronic diseases like diabetes, hypertension, respiratory diseases, etc.

Patients may come for immediate admission and treatment in cases of heart attack, poisoning, fits, animal bites, injuries, accidents, paralysis, diarrhea, fevers, labor pains, asthma, unconsciousness, shock, etc. Indoor paper is prepared in outpatient department (OPD) or casualty, stat orders are written, emergency treatment is carried out in casualty or in minor operation theater (OT) or patient is sent to concerned ward. Patient received in ambulance should be transferred on stretcher. Patient should not be left alone but always accompanied by nurse or trained person. A female patient should never be kept alone with male attendant.

Receiving in Ward

Nurse admitting patient should receive patient and relative with greet, friendliness, smile and establish an effective nurse-patient relationship. If patient is very ill, put to bed immediately. Relatives are treated with courtesy. Walking patients may go around and they may be oriented with the ward environment. Explain hospital policies, procedures, routines and what is expected of him. Relatives may be allowed to stay till patient is comfortable. Patient on self-diet is to be explained about type of diet to be taken and hours at which it can be brought to ward.

Helping the Patient to Bed

Closed bed is converted to open bed. Transfer from stretcher or wheel chair to bed or patient can walk into bed. Make him or her comfortable and monitor temperature, pulse, aspirations and record the time and prepare the temperature chart, writing ward number, bed number, patient's name, age, sex, date and time of admission and record temperature, pulse, respiration (TPR). If stat orders are to be carried out, carry out those orders and record on chart. Give clean clothes and assist for changing, if needed. Give comfortable position as per need. If patient's condition permits and he needs, bed bath may be given. Patient can be observed for injuries, rash, infection, pediculosis, discharge from body, full bladder, swelling, oral hygiene and mental status.

Collect specimens of urine, stool, blood. Clothes should be sent with relatives for washing, otherwise they are numbered, labeled and kept in store. If infected, disinfection is needed. Encourage patient to send his or her jewelery and valuables. Negligence in handling patient's belongings brings blame on hospital and personnel working and patients become suspicious and create a bad image. Valuables can be returned to patient or relative and get receipt when patient is discharged. In case of patient's death handover the belongings to relative and obtain receipt of it. In medicolegal cases preservation of clothes is legal responsibility as it may be used as evidence in court of law. Clothes and belongings of such patients should be kept in safe custody. After admission, patient's name, address, age, sex, date and time of admission, phone number is entered in admission book. If record is computerized it can be entered in computer. Monitor patient's condition and enter in nurse's notes and in patient's case paper.

Special Considerations

Check vital signs, level of consciousness, observe for wound, hemorrhage, fracture, dehydration, fever, and hypothermia, be quick. Check and decide to assist physician or surgeon with necessary equipment. Give cardiopulmonary resuscitation (CPR), if required. Casualty medical officer is always there to assess client's condition. Quick assistance is needed. It is responsibility of a nurse to see all the equipment are in working order and emergency drugs, equipment, syringes, needles, IV fluids, oxygen is available.

Medicolegal Cases

Cases of accidents, poisoning, burns, suicidal and homicidal attempts, drug abuse, sex abuse are considered as medicolegal cases. Recording of date and time of admission, assessment by physician or surgeon, saving of specimens, body tissues, clothes, signing of documents and notifying police is must, which will serve as evidence in court of law.

Role and Responsibilities of a Nurse

Nurse uses her clinical judgment in giving care, admitting and transferring patient to a particular ward or department. She assists physician and surgeon in giving emergency care. She sees to the comfort of the patient in routine admission. She orients patient to the ward and carries out physician's orders intelligently and immediately. She records all observations made date, time, vitals, and drugs given. She arranges for investigations, diet, and treatment. She explains relatives about patient's condition, takes consent, if required, and explains rules, regulations and other procedures. She arranges teaching, if needed for patients and relatives. She explains about surgical treatment, other requirements, blood, intravenous fluids, drugs, if to be arranged. If child mother or father stays with child, she explains to parents about child and care to be taken.

DISCHARGE PLANNING

Begin discharge planning at the time of admission or even before the admission, in cases of same day surgery or childbirth. Assess client's condition and involve client and family in discharge planning process.
Prepare discharge summary: It consists of client's unresolved problems and continued health care, reason for hospitalization, significant findings, client's status and specific teaching plan. Prepare discharge card with clear, concise description in client's own language. Step-by-step description of procedure to be performed. Precautions to follow for self-care and medicine to be taken, e.g. taking insulin, skin care, diet restrictions. Review signs and symptoms and report to physician. List phone numbers of healthcare providers and resources to contact. Identify unresolved. Inform police, if medicolegal case, and send papers to police *chouki* for sign. Check the doctor's orders for discharge and discharge notes and card. Give instructions for follow-up, OPD days, when to come. Check articles which were given to him, confirm he has paid all the bills. List

actual time of discharge, mode of transportation, who accompanied the client. Record, in the admission, discharge book, Giraffe omnibed (GOB), the date and time of discharge. Set the unit for new patient. If patient was infectious, disinfection of articles, carbolization or fumigation should be done. Disinfect and send linen to laundry.

Role and Responsibility of Nurse

- Participate in discharge planning procedure with physician, patient, and relatives
- Check the physician's order for discharge
- Note the type of discharge on medical advice, against medical advice, absconded, etc.
- Inform police, if medicolegal case or absconded
- Document date and time of discharge
- Hand over patient's belongings obtaining receipt
- Ensure bills are paid
- Give instructions regarding follow-up, special care at home, diet, etc.

Care of the Patient's Unit After Discharge

Clean, disinfect, and sterilize the equipment such as trays, bowls, bedpan, urinal, etc. Send linen to laundry. If linen is infected, send for washing after disinfecting. Wipe mattress with wet cloth and dry in sun, or if there is facility autoclave. Clean the furniture in room. Make a bed with clean linen. Keep necessary articles near bed that is drinking water in jug, glass, bedpan and urinal.

TRANSFER OF PATIENT

Patient may be transferred from one department of the hospital to the other or to other hospital. Doctor writes the order of transfer in consultation with other department. Incharge sister is informed as she makes the arrangements to receive the patient in her ward. Patient's belongings, complete case paper with charts, reports, X-rays, should be sent along with. Patient should be transferred on wheel chair or stretcher and accompanied by nurse. Patient and relatives are to be explained the purpose behind the transfer. Record in the admission book, transfer book, GOB, transfer of patient. When the transfer is made to other hospital, correspondence is made by the department to that hospital prior to transfer or relatives make arrangements in other hospital for admission and procedure is as for discharge of patient and it is mentioned where patient is sent.

TYPES OF DISCHARGE

Discharge from Postanesthetic Care Unit

Postanesthesia recovery score is used for assessment (score of 8–10) before discharge. If below 4, surgeon transfers patient to ICU. Communication occurs between postanesthetic care unit (PACU) nurse and the nurse on nursing unit. This includes vital signs, type of surgery, anesthesia used, blood loss, level of consciousness (LOC), general physical condition, IV lines, drainage tubes and dressings. Patient is transferred on stretcher.

Interdisciplinary Discharge

Discharge to acute rehabilitation, skilled nursing, home and adult home.

Discharge instructions regarding body weight, diet restrictions, care to be taken, advice is written. Medications, dose purpose, time to be taken, special instructions, when to come or see doctor is written.

Discharge Against Medical Advice

Patient goes home even when doctor has not advised discharge. He goes on his own risk giving written information on case paper with time and date written.

Absconding

Patient leaves the unit without giving any information.

Leaving Against Medical Advice (LAMA)

Occasionally, patient or family may demand discharge against medical advice. If this occurs, notify physician immediately. He will ask the patient to sign a form against medical advice (AMA) releasing the facility from legal responsibility for any medical problems patient may experience after discharge. If physician is not available discuss the form with patient and obtain signature. Do not detain the patient. After the patient leaves, document the incidence thoroughly in your notes and notify physician.

DISCHARGE SUMMARY

Discharge summary or referral summary are completed when patient is being discharged and referred to another institution or to home. A narrative discharge summary in the progress note includes:

- Client's status on admission and discharge or referral
- A brief summary of client care
- Interventions and education outcome
- Resolved problems and continuing care needs, unresolved problems including referrals
- Patient's instructions about medications, diet, food-drug interactions, activity, treatments, follow-up and other special needs.

CHAPTER

4

Communications and Nurse-Patient Relationship

AIM

Students know the basic communication skills and are able to put in to practice.

OBJECTIVES

- Students are able to communicate with patients, relatives, coworkers, and superiors
- Students are able to write nurse's notes, records and reports
- Students are able to interview clients.

COMMUNICATION

Definition

Communication is a process of sending and receiving information, ideas, feelings or encoding and decoding of information.

Importance of Good Communication

Communication is the means of establishing helping and healing relationships. Caring nurse communicate with others in manner that expresses awareness and respect for persons as individuals, with knowledge and consideration of their specific needs. It develops help, trust relationship and nurse-client relationship. Good interpersonal communication and responding appropriately develop a sense of mutuality. All communications contain stimuli to influence others. Nurse's communication can result in harm or good. Good communication empowers others and enable people to know themselves and make their own choices, an essential part of healing process. Communication helps to reduce interpersonal tensions, improve interpersonal relationships in health team. It helps nurse to understand patient, inform relatives, superiors and coworkers. It will help her to influence behavior of those whom she deals with. It also helps to interpret the hospital policies and patient care.

Elements of Communication (Table 4.1)

There are four major elements of communication:

1. Source
2. Message
3. Channel
4. Receiver.

Source or Sender

From where ideas or purposes are perceived to be communicated to receiver to produce desired responses. Making use of intellectual capacities, speaking, writing, drawing and demonstrating ability to achieve desired response. Sender encodes the message.

Message

Ideas, purpose or intended goals and objectives, information and facts.

Channel

Channel is the medium of communication which helps to transmit message from source to receiver.

Table 4.1: Elements of communication

Source or Sender	*Message*	*Channel*	*Receiver*
• Perceives ideas, purpose goals and objectives	• Produce desired results	• Speech—vocal mechanism • Sound waves • Written words • Drawings, pictures • Body language • Audiovisual aids • Electronic media	• Receives message • Decodes message

Receiver

Receiver receives message through channel sent by sender and decodes it.

Face-to-Face Communication

Oral message, spoken words are transmitted through vocal mechanism and sound waves. Nonverbal messages are transmitted by written words, pictures, body language that is gestures, posture, facial expressions. Audio-visual aids such as radio, TV, printed material, projected aids.

Receiver

Any person for whom message is intended. Receiver receives message and decodes it. Listening, reading, writing, interpreting, judging and responding.

Types of Communications

- Verbal
- Nonverbal
- Written.

Verbal Communication

The word spoken is mode of communication for conveying information, ideas, thoughts and feelings. Use of spoken words is verbal communication. Sender sends message, encoding in words and receiver converts it to thoughts, ideas. If the transmission process is accurate, ideas of sender and receiver are same. If they differ, it is break in communication. Telephone, message, face-to-face talk are examples of verbal communication.

Nonverbal Communication

Gestures, facial expressions, body postures, body movements, actions are forms of nonverbal communication. Crying, laughing, dilated pupils, smiling, hand locking, clenching fists, frowning, grimace, holding of body parts for pain, movements of hands and fingers, lips also help in nonverbal communication. Greeting, hugging express love and affection. Pain, joy, anger, love, sorrow can be expressed by nonverbal communication. Role play method of health education is example of nonverbal communication. Touch can express many feelings. Stroking back, wiping tears, tapping shoulders communicate empathy. Keeping hand on forehead, listening to complaints are some of the examples of nonverbal communication. Keeping index finger on lips is symbol for keeping silence, raising eyebrows questioning, moving head, nodding are also body languages.

Written Communication

Notes on patient's history of illness, physical examination, order of medicine and injection, treatment reports, care plans, records, letters are types of written communication.

Lines of Communication

- Intrapersonal
- Interpersonal.

Intrapersonal

Occurring within an individual. Self-talk, self-instructions, inner thoughts, or inner dialogue. Positive self-talk can be used as a tool to improve nurse's and client's health and self-esteem. Self-instructions can be useful for difficult tasks or situations and are also useful to develop self-awareness, positive self-concept and self-expression.

Interpersonal

One-to-one interaction. It takes place within social context. It includes all symbols and cues. It helps in exchange of ideas, goal accomplishment, team building, and personal growth. Small group communication when small number of people meet together helps to understand group dynamics. It produces cohesiveness and commitment.

Channels of Communication

Channels are means of conveying and receiving messages through visual, auditory and tactile senses. Spoken and written words, facial expressions touch, telephone, pager, VCD, Fax, e-mail, internet are means of communication.

Methods of Effective Communication

- Attending skills
- Rapport building skills
- Empathy skills.

Attending Skills

Active listening. Be attentive to what patient says verbally and nonverbally. Sit facing the patient. It is nonverbal communication that you are interested in what patient says.

- Observe an open posture. Do not lock hands and legs
- Lean towards patient
- Establish and maintain eye contact
- Relax.

Rapport Building Skills

Observe, focus onto messages conveyed. Restate his message briefly in own words (paraphrasing), ask relevant questions. One question at a time and exploring one topic fully before going to next. Do not give personal opinion. Avoid personal questions. Do not give false assurance.

Empathy Skills

Empathy is ability to understand and accept another person's reality, to perceive feelings and to communicate this feeling to others. Nurse has to be sensitive and imaginative. Empathy statements are neutral and nonjudgmental used to develop trust. She shares hope with patient. Encouragement and positive feedback are important for fostering hope and self-confidence. Sharing humor, feelings, using touch, using silence, providing information, clarifying, focusing, paraphrasing helps to build rapport.

Factors Affecting Communication

- Knowledge—knowledge about facts
- Skill—communication skill, pacing, intonation, clarity and brevity
- Attitude—attitude of sender and receiver, timings and relevance
- Position in sociocultural system
- Factors related to message
- Factors related to channel
- Characterization of speech
- Use of body language
- Condition of vocal mechanism
- Characteristics of written words, drawing
- Type and nature of audiovisual aids

- Receiver's ability and level of knowledge
- Receiver's readiness and motivation
- Physical and social environment.

Barriers of Communication

- Defective senses—speech, hearing, sight
- Language, educational level, customs
- Physical inability to convey or receive message
- Power failure
- Dead phones
- Media failure
- Pain, hunger, weakness, fatigue, dyspnea
- Developmental factors
- Emotional factors—fear, anger, jealousy, suspicion, grief, prejudice, lack of interest in listening.

Methods to Improve Communication

Professional is expected to be clean, neat, well-groomed, conservatively dressed, scent and odor free. Professional appearance and behavior are important in establishing trustworthiness and competence. Professional behavior should reflect warmth, friendliness, confidence and competence. Being on time, organized, well-prepared and equipped for responsibilities of nursing role will communicate professionalism. Using names and acknowledging client, making eye contact, smiling and not calling clients by bed numbers or diagnosis as identification. Maintaining proper record system, writing accurate correct records and reports, maintenance of equipment of communication, group discussions, conferences, improving interpersonal relationships, and teamwork will improve communication.

HELPING RELATIONSHIP: NURSE-PATIENT RELATIONSHIP

Dimensions and Phases of NPR

Helping relationships are basis of clinical nursing practice. Nurse is a professional helper and knows the client as an individual, who has unique health needs, pattern of living, and human response. The relationship is therapeutic, promoting a psychological climate that helps positive change and growth. Nurse uses therapeutic communication for patients to achieve expected outcomes for optimum health. It is confidential, goal directed and within time frame. Nurse establishes, directs and interacts, taking patient's needs as priority. Nurse accepts patient without judgment. She hears messages or acknowledges feelings. Nurse-patient relationship is created with care, skill and is built on patient's trust in nurse.

Therapeutic Communication Phases

- Preinteraction
- Orientation
- Working phase
- Termination phase.

Preinteraction

Socializing: It is initial component of interpersonal relationship. It helps to know each other and relax. It is easy, superficial and not deeply personal.

Orientation

Nurse's introduction. Explain why data is collected. Assure confidentiality. Sign authorization referring to hospital policy. Establish trust and confidence. Be aware that the client is forming impression about nursing. It is new experience for him. Client should feel comfortable as the orientation phase proceeds. Use professionalism and competence. Nurse's attitude, professional manner, appearance, encourage supportive therapeutic relationship.

Working Phase

Nurse gathers information about client's health status. Nurse uses interview technique, asking questions to gather complete data. She uses technique of listening, paraphrasing, focusing, summarizing and clarifying to facilitate communication.

Termination Phase

Clue is given that interview is coming to an end. Summarize important points, ask his opinion about accuracy of it. Terminate interview in friendly manner.

Communicating effectively with patients, families, team members and maintain effective human relations. When communicating with families, the same principles of patient helping relationship apply, but in family additional understanding of family dynamics, needs, relationships are to be taken into consideration.

Relationship with team members needs team building, group process, collaborative consultation, delegation, supervision, leadership and management.

Everyone has interpersonal need for acceptance, inclusions, identity, privacy, power and control, and affection. Nurses need friendship, support, guidance, encouragement from others to cope with stressors and she also must extend some caring communication used with clients to build positive relationship with coworkers.

COMMUNICATION IN VULNERABLE GROUP

Clients Who are Cognitively Impaired

- Reduce environmental distractions while conversing
- Get clients's attention prior to speaking
- Use simple sentences
- Avoid long explanations
- Ask one question at a time
- Allow time for client to respond
- Be an attentive listener
- Include family and friends in conversation, especially in subject known to client.

Clients Who Cannot Speak Clearly

- Listen attentively, be patient and do not interrupt
- Ask simple questions that require "Yes", "No" answers
- Allow time for understanding and response
- Don not shout or speak loudly
- Encourage the client to speak
- Let client know, if you have not understood
- Use visual aids
- Use communication aids, e.g. pad and pen
- Use nonverbal communication.

Patient Teaching

Importance

Nurses are responsible to teach their patients. Patients have right to information about their care. Patients and their families often ask for health information.

Purpose

- To acquire new knowledge, attitude, behavior and skills
- To assess the needs
- To establish interpersonal communication.

Process

- Nurse perceives the need to provide information, establishes relevant learning objectives
- She performs activities aimed at helping patient and family to learn
- She sends information about knowledge of teaching content, teaching approach, experience, emotions and values
- Channels she uses are methods used to present content, e.g. Aids.

ROLE OF NURSE AND INTEGRATING TEACHING IN NURSING PROCESS

- Develop learning objectives
- Set priorities, timings
- Maintain learning attention and participation
- Nurse individualizes the teaching plan
- Select teaching method
- Tell, sell, participate, entrust and reinforce
- Discuss, demonstrate, stimulate, speak in their language, and use teaching tools
- Document the teaching.

CHAPTER

5

The Nursing Process

AIM

Students use nursing process in patient care.

OBJECTIVES

- Students explain the concept, uses, format and steps of nursing process
- Students document nursing process as per the format.

CRITICAL THINKING AND NURSING JUDGMENT

Components

- Specific knowledge base in nursing
- Experience in nursing
- **Critical thinking competencies:** This includes general and specific critical competencies in clinical setting
- **Attitude for critical thinking:** Confidence, independence, fairness, responsibility, risk taking, discipline, perseverance, creativity, curiosity, integrity and humility
- **Standards for critical thinking:** There are intellectual and professional standards for critical thinking. Intellectual standards are clear, precise, specific, accurate, relevant, plausible, consistent, logical, deep, broad, complete, significant, adequate and fair. Professional standards are ethical criteria for nursing judgment, criteria for evaluation and professional responsibility.

Nurses specific knowledge base depends upon educational qualification, continuing education, reading, knowledge of basic science and ability to think critically about health problems. Clinical experience given opportunity implement theoretical knowledge in practice. She understands clinical situations. All clinical experience are stepping stones for building new knowledge. Based upon nursing knowledge, experience and the above said attitudes, she is able to make nursing judgments.

Critical Thinking

Thinking and learning is a lifelong process. New knowledge, refining ability to think, problem solving, making judgment are helpful for intellectual and emotional growth. There are always new things coming up, as nursing science advances and are to be applied in practice. Learning effective, scientific, relevant interventions will result in better outcomes. Learning makes nurses think critically and positively.

Critical thinking competencies are the cognitive processes used for nursing judgments (Flowchart 5.1).

Competencies, Attitude for Critical Thinking

General Competencies

- General critical thinking
- Specific critical thinking in clinical situation
- Specific critical thinking in nursing.

General Critical Thinking

- Scientific method
- Problem-solving
- Decision-making.

Flowchart 5.1: Critical thinking

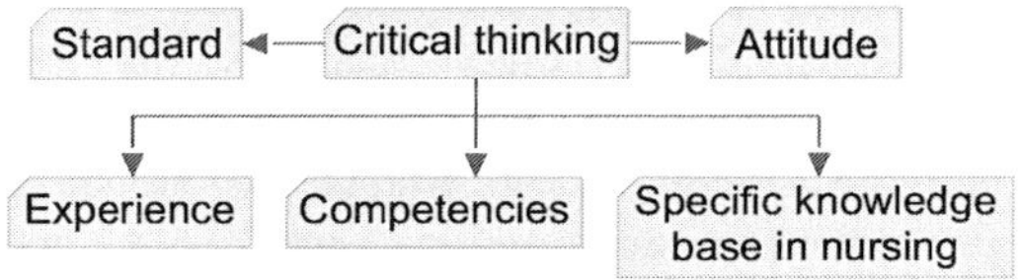

Specific Critical Thinking in Clinical Situation

- Diagnostic reasoning
- Clinical inference
- Clinical decision-making.

Specific Critical Thinking in Nursing Application of Nursing Process

- **Scientific method:** It is an approach to find out truth or verifying the set facts which agree with reality. Example—Research method
- **Problem-solving:** When problem arises we find solution by obtaining information and adding what we already know. It also evaluates solution over time to be sure that it is still effective
- **Decision-making:** It is end point of critical thinking that leads to problem solution. It involves following steps like assessing options, testing option, considering consequences and making decision
  - **Diagnostic reasoning:** Forming a nursing diagnosis based on information gathered.
  - **Informing:** Drawing conclusion from data obtained
  - **Clinical decision-making:** Choosing nursing intervention requires reasoning.

LEVELS OF CRITICAL THINKING

- Basic critical thinking
- Complex critical thinking
- Commitment.

Basic Critical Thinking

Learner trusts experts thinking is concrete and based on set of rules or principles, e.g. use of procedures, manuals.

Complex Critical Thinking

Learner analyzes and examines alternatives more independently.

Thinking abilities and initiative makes learner to look beyond expert opinions. Each solution has benefits and risks.

Commitment

Learner takes responsibility, makes choice without assistance from others, and assumes accountability for it.

NURSING PROCESS

Definition

Nursing process is an orderly, systematic study for identifying patient's health problems and making plans to solve them, initiating the plans or assigning others to implement it and evaluating the extent to which the plan was effective in solving the problems identified.

Step I: Nursing assessment
- Data gathering
  - Subjective—history, patient's complaints, feelings
  - Objective—findings of physical examination and laboratory reports.

Step II: Making nursing diagnosis.
Step III: Writing outcome/Goal Statements/objectives.
Step IV: Determining appropriate nursing interventions.
Step V: Implementing nursing care.
Step VI: Evaluating nursing care.

Step I: Assessment—history—subjective data.
Physical examination—objective data.
Review of laboratory reports—objective data.
Step II: Nursing diagnosis—clinical judgment about response to health problem.

- **Cues**—subjective or objective data, cluster of signs and symptoms or behavior
- **Inference**—giving meaning to cues.
- **Related factors**—situation, conditions contributing to nursing diagnosis.
  For example, high risk for aspiration related to excessive oral secretion.
  Altered body temperature related to hyperthermia.

Step III: Writing outcome/goal.
For example, patient maintains normal body temperature, patient maintains patient airway.

Step IV: Determining nursing intervention

- Setting priorities
- Developing specific outcomes
- Verification of outcomes
- Identifying interventions and time frame.

ASSESSMENT, COLLECTION OF DATA, TYPES, SOURCES, METHODS

It is continuous as part of nursing process as basis to plan a care. Continuous assessment for nursing diagnosis and selecting intervention is necessary. First, assessment on admission is made in detail to obtain all basic information. Further assessment is made to evaluate the implemented nursing care plan. Reassessment to make appropriate changes in care plan.

For example, patient with altered body temperature related to disease condition, hyperthermia. Hydrotherapy and other care is given according to plan.

To evaluate the effectiveness of care, assessment is made, e.g. check body temperature, pulse, observe sweating, peripheral circulation, general condition of the patient. Care plans will change according to assessments. Patient may develop certain problems during the hospital stay. Therapy, surgery, medications will change condition of patient unless he is assessed for changes cannot be noted. It is important for documentation and reporting as the whole care depends on assessment.

FORMULATING NURSING JUDGMENT: DATA INTERPRETATION

Analysis and interpretation of data assessment requires critical thinking. Nurse validates the collected information to ensure its accuracy. Comparison is made with another source; nurse may ask patient or family member for validation of information obtained in health history. Additions and corrections are noted. Data in medical record, consultation with other health team members is of help to validate the observation and physical assessment data. Through process of inferential reasoning and judgment nurse interprets the data.

Data clustering: After validation and interpreting assessment data, nurse organizes the information into meaningful clusters. Cluster is a set of signs and symptoms. Cues help to generate nursing diagrams, e.g. pain, anxiety, immobility.

Assess and reassess: Validate data with client and family, interpret and analyzes, cluster the data (group signs and symptoms), classify and organize and begin formulating nursing diagnosis, e.g. in patient's history information collected is low economic group, habit of consuming alcohol, poor diet. In physical assessment, it is found edema over feet, increased abdominal girth, nutritional deficiency signs, anxiety, dyspnea.

When clustering the information patients self-care ability is also assessed. The diagnosis may be altered, nutritional status less than body requirement. Risk for pressure ulcer related to edema, emaciation. Altered respiratory pattern related to abdominal distension. Altered mobility related to edema, abdominal distension.

NURSING DIAGNOSIS

Nursing diagnosis relates to specific health problems or responses to disease process or treatment and nursing interventions. It is a clinical judgment about individual, family or community responses to actual or potential health problems/life processes. Cues are subjective or objective data collected from assessment. Diagnostic cues are clusters of signs and symptoms or behaviors. They are measurable through observation and record.

Inferencing: Giving meaning to cues

Defining diagnosis: These are manifestations

(Clinical cues that cluster as manifestations)

Related factors: Situations, conditions that can cause or contribute to nursing diagnosis. These factors can be physical, physiological, environmental and psychological.

Diagnosis

- High risk for injury related to change in mental status or excessive fatigue and altered gait
- High risk for aspiration related to excessive oral secretions
- Fatigue related to persistent shortness of breath
- Feeding self-care deficit related to pain in fingers.

DIFFERENCE BETWEEN MEDICAL DIAGNOSIS AND NURSING DIAGNOSIS

Medical diagnosis is identifying disease condition on the basis of physical signs, symptoms, history and result of diagnostic tests. Physician gives treatment for the condition diagnosed by medicines and therapies and surgeon operates and removes abnormal part of the body or reconstruction of body tissues. Nursing diagnosis is to identify or to know the responses to actual or potential health problems or life processes judged clinically for the patient, family or community. It is statement that describes the patient's actual or potential response to health problem that nurse is licensed and competent to treat. Impaired skin integrity, risk of infection, fluid volume deficit, knowledge deficit, low self-esteem are some of the examples of nursing diagnosis statement. Nursing diagnosis provides the basis for selection of nursing interventions to achieve outcomes for which the nurse in responsible.

Planning

- Setting priorities
- Developing specific outcomes
- Verification of outcomes
- Identifying nursing interventions and time frame.

Setting Priority

- **High priority:** Life-threatening nursing diagnosis requiring immediate actions, e.g. tissue perfusion, risk for aspiration, ineffective airway clearance
- **Medium priority:** Problems are not life-threatening, but may result in physical or psychological consequences, e.g. impaired physical mobility leading to contracture, pneumonia, depression, etc.
- **Low priority:** Those problems which person can handle with minimal assistance, e.g. self-esteem, self-actualization, altered body image.

  Planning, establishing goals and expected outcomes. Once the nursing diagnosis is identified for the patient think about the best approach to solve the problems (Table 5.1).

Table 5.1: Setting priorities to determine nursing intervention

High	*Medium*	*Low*
Life-threatening situations, e.g. • Risk for aspiration • Airway clearance • Tissue perfusion altered	Problem not life-threatening but may result in physical or psychological consequences, e.g. • Immobility risk for pressure sore • Risk for oral infection	Problem requiring minimal assistance, e.g. • Low self-esteem • Self-actualization • Altered body image

Goals and expected outcomes are specific statements of patient's behavior or physiological responses that nurse sets to achieve problem solution, e.g. client will sit and stand by evening on first postoperative day. Client will achieve normal fluid volume. It provides direction for selection of nursing intervention.

For example, to achieve first expected outcome nursing interventions are turning, change of position, early ambulation, encouragement and motivation. It also helps in evaluation and modifying the plan. Expected outcomes are specific measurable changes in patient's status that is expected to occur in response to nursing care.

Selecting Interventions

When selecting intervention six factors are to be thought of. Type of nursing diagnosis, expected outcomes, research base, feasibility of intervention, acceptability to patient, competencies of nurse. Review standardized care plans, NIC, critical pathways, policy procedure manuals, textbooks, nursing literature and collaboration.

Developing Specific Outcomes

To develop specific outcomes taking into consideration, the physiological status, psychological status, functioned measures, knowledge, symptom control, safety is a need.

Verifying Outcomes

Outcome is measurable, observable change in person's health status. They must be clear, concise, client centered, specific and measurable. Use terms administers, demonstrates, has increase in or decrease in, states, performs, identifies, etc. For example, patient is able to expectorate secretions effectively. Breath sounds within normal limits within 72 hours.

Identifying Nursing Intervention and Time Frame

Setting time frame: It is deadline to accomplish outcome. Specifying the date for outcome. Reflects the judgment about the time needed. Judgment is based upon your knowledge, about health problem, client's condition, support system and nursing interventions. It requires critical thinking.

Identifying Nursing Interventions

Nursing interventions are nursing actions, activities, approaches and orders. Types—Independent and Interdependent.

Independent interventions depend on nursing diagnosis. These actions do not require physician's orders. Nurses are qualified to carry them out independently by law and educational preparation. Interdependant interventions are those performed by nurses in collaboration with other members of the team, e.g. physician, dietician, physiotherapist, occupational therapist, etc.

Independent nursing interventions include such actions as counseling, teaching, mouth care, relaxation training, bathing, changing position, feeding, assisting with ambulation while interdependant nursing interventions include administration of medicine, dressing, administration of IV fluids, drawing blood, obtaining specimens. Other interventions include answering phone, bed making, serving trays and obtaining equipments.

Implementation

It is a fourth step of nursing process, begins after the care plan is developed. Nurse initiates the intervention, planned to support or improve client's health status. It is implemented according to need, situation. In this step, nurse provides care to patients. She completes the action or interventions to achieve goal or expected outcome. Direct care interventions are treatments performed through interaction with patient. Indirect care implies care of the environment likes safety, infection control, documentation, co-ordination. Implementation is continuous process according to patient's condition. Response to interventions is evaluated and again assessment is made to identify needs. Knowledge of nursing interventions, intervention skills helps nurse in implementation. Implementation involves critical thinking in choosing interventions, e.g. expected outcome, nursing diagnosis, evidence base for interventions, feasibility of performing, acceptability and nurse's capability.

Evaluation

It is final step of nursing process. Nurse checks expected outcome, which are standard to check effectiveness of intervention. Positive evaluation occurs when desired results are met. Use of evaluative measures through assessment skill is made and decisions are made about progress and patient's status.

Documentation and Reporting

These are part of evaluation process. Accurate record of client's status, decisions made by nurses are recorded. All objective data should be documented using appropriate measurements and details. Nurses notes, assessment sheets, sharing of information, change of shift reports should communicate patient's progress and outcomes and goal of nursing care.

Protocols and Standing Orders

Protocol is a written plan specifying the procedure to be followed during care of patients with selected clinical conditions or situation, e.g. post-operative patient protocol provides standard of care or clinical guideline which can be individualized for specific client. Protocol can be used strictly within the framework of independent nursing intervention, e.g. admission, discharge, pain management, CPR, and other therapies like speech therapy, occupational therapy and physiotherapy.

Standing order is carried out until the prescriber cancels it by another order or until a prescribed number of days elapse. Standing order may indicate a final date, a number of treatments or doses.

For example, "decadron 10 mg daily × 5 days, standing order is preprinted document containing orders for the conduct of routine therapies, monitoring guidelines and or diagnostic procedures for specific clients with identified clinical problem.

Standing orders are commonly formed in critical care settings, community health settings. These orders give legal protection to nurses to intervene appropriately in clients best interest.

Application in Practice and Implications

Speak confidently. Be certain of being able to perform care safely. Always be prepared before performing nursing activity. Share ideas about nursing interventions with colleagues. Listen to both sides in any discussions. Ask for help, if you are not sure. Report any problem immediately. Follow standards of practice in patient care. Be thorough with whatever you do. Use scientific and practice based criteria for activities. Specific knowledge base, experience, confidence, thinking independently, responsibility and accountability, risk taking, discipline and perseverance, creativity, curiosity, integrity, humility are important factors in critical thinking which makes a nurse possible to make judgments and apply into practice.

NURSING CARE PLAN

It is written plan that states nursing diagnosis, outcomes and nursing intervention. It provides detailed guide for nursing care, individualizes nursing care, provides source of information, fosters continuity of care, outlines discharge program and coordinates team effort. It reflects current nursing practice.

Writing nursing care plan, implementation evaluation—outcome of care—review and modify. Nursing care plan is guide for clinical care. It serves as a document that communicates patient's nursing care to all members of health team.

Nursing care plan and nursing process formats are given in table 5.2 and 5.3.

Types

Student's care plans, institutional care plans and concept maps.

Purpose

- To direct clinical care
- To decrease risk of incompleteness
- To identify quickly nursing diagnosis, expected outcome and nursing intervention to be done
- To coordinate nursing care by all the members
- To schedule diagnostic tests

Table 5.2: Nursing Care Plan Format

Assessment	*Nursing diagnosis*	*Goal*	*Intervention*	*Rationale*	*Implementation*	*Evaluation*
1	2	3	4	5	6	7

Table 5.3: Nursing Process Format

Assessment	*Nursing diagnosis*	*Goal*	*Nursing intervention planned*	*Nursing intervention implemented*	*Outcome/ Result*
• Dyspnea • Cyanosis	• Impaired breathing • Altered tissue perfusion	• Breathing improves • Tissues receive sufficient oxygen	Propped up position loosen clothing, O_2 therapy	Fowler's position given support with extra pillows cardiac table O_2 inhalation started 4 lit/mm	Cyanosis disappeared No dyspnea, tissue perfusion improved

Table 5.4: Students care plans

Nursing assessment	*Nursing diagnosis*	*Rationale*	*Goal/ outcome*	*Rationale*	*Nursing intervention planned*	*Rationale*	*Nursing intervention implemented*	*Evaluation*
1	2	3	4	5	6	7	8	9

- To identify and coordinate resources
- To enhance continuity of care
- To organize information exchanged by nurses when change of shift
- To focus reports on nursing care and treatment
- Includes long-term goals
- Family is involved
- Helps to evaluate, provides direction for implementation and framework of education.

Student's Care Plans

Students learn problem-solving technique as part of their education. The plan format is given in table 5.4

Institutional Care Plans

Institutional care plans are concise documents that become part of the client's medical record.

- **Kardex nursing care plan:** It is trade name for card filling system that allows quick reference to the particular needs of the client for certain aspects of nursing care. Medications, activity levels, level of self-care diet, treatment and procedures. Each institution has its own format for kardex
- **Computerized care plans:** Prewritten plans created for specific nursing diagnosis, e.g. immobility, abdominal surgery, postpartum care
- **Critical pathways:** It is integrated care plan for projected length by health team. It shows day-by-day client's activities, consults, procedures, discharge planning, education topics. It shows responsibility of individual person. It shows evidence-based protocols for specific cases
- **Concept maps:** It is a tool that assists learner in developing self-appraisal. It is diagram of client's problems and interventions relationship, use of concept map promotes critical thinking and helps student to organize complex data.

CHAPTER

6

Documentation and Reporting

AIM

Students know how to document and report.

OBJECTIVES

- Students understand importance of documentation
- Students are able to document and report.

DOCUMENTATION AND REPORTING

Documentation is written or printed that is relied on as a record or proof for authorized person.

Purpose of Documentation and Reporting

- It is valuable source of data, used by all members of health team
- It is confidential, permanent legal document of information related to patient care
- It is useful for legal claims
- It is used for education and research
- Statements can be used as evidence
- It is written, relied upon and proof for authorized persons
- It is comprehensive, purposive, accurate, providing detailed account of level of quality care delivered to patients
- It saves time, minimizes errors and ensures continuity of care
- It communicates information in timely and effective manner

- Communicating within healthcare team patients records and report are for effective communication within healthcare team.

Records and Reports are Written Communications

- Patient's case record: Case paper, contains ward number, bed number, name, sex, age, address, date and time of admission, provisional diagnosis, treatment and observations, laboratory reports, X-ray reports, operation notes, pre- and postoperative order, treatment and consent
- Charts: Temperature chart (Flowchart 6.1), pulse and blood pressure record, intake and output chart (Table 6.1), level of consciousness (LOC) chart
- Admission record, nursing care plans, nurses notes
- Discharge record, teaching on discharge
- Treatment record, follow-up instructions
- Stock and issue register, medicine account
- Inventory, day report, night report
- Bed list, record of admission, discharge, death, transfer
- Death record
- Specimen book, doctor's call book, autoclave book, laundry book, diet book
- Duty list, work distribution.

Each record communicates about particular event and information to others.

NURSES NOTES (TABLE 6.2)

Notes written by nurses regarding nursing interventions performed and evaluation based on nursing assessment, diagnosis, interventions are planned and implemented. Every intervention has rationale behind. After completing the intervention, she has to record and write on nurses notes. It includes date, time, nursing action, result, and signature. She is responsible and accountable for interventions and writing those intervention in nurses notes.

Ward No:	Bed No:	Patient's Name:	Age:
Sex:	Date:	Time:	Notes:

Record must contain descriptive and objective information about what a nurse sees, hears, feels, and smells.

Flowchart 6.1: Temperature chart

Ward No:	**Diagnosis:** Upper respiratory Infection (URI)	**Bed No:**
Female Medical Ward		**Reg. No:**
Date of Adm:		**Patient's Name:**
Time of Adm:		**Age: , Sex:**

Month	March															
Date	22			23			24			25			26	27	28	C
Time F	2/6	10/6	6/10	2/6	10/2	6/10	2/6	10/2	6/10	2/6	10/2	6/10	6/6	6/6	6/6	
160 106																42
150 105																
140 104																41
130 103																40
120 102																
110 101																39
100 100																38
90 99																
80 98																37
70 97																36
60 96																
50 95																35
P T Resp		24/20	20/20	28/16	16/16	20/20	20/16	16/16	16/16	20/20	20/20	20/20	16/16	16/16	16/16	

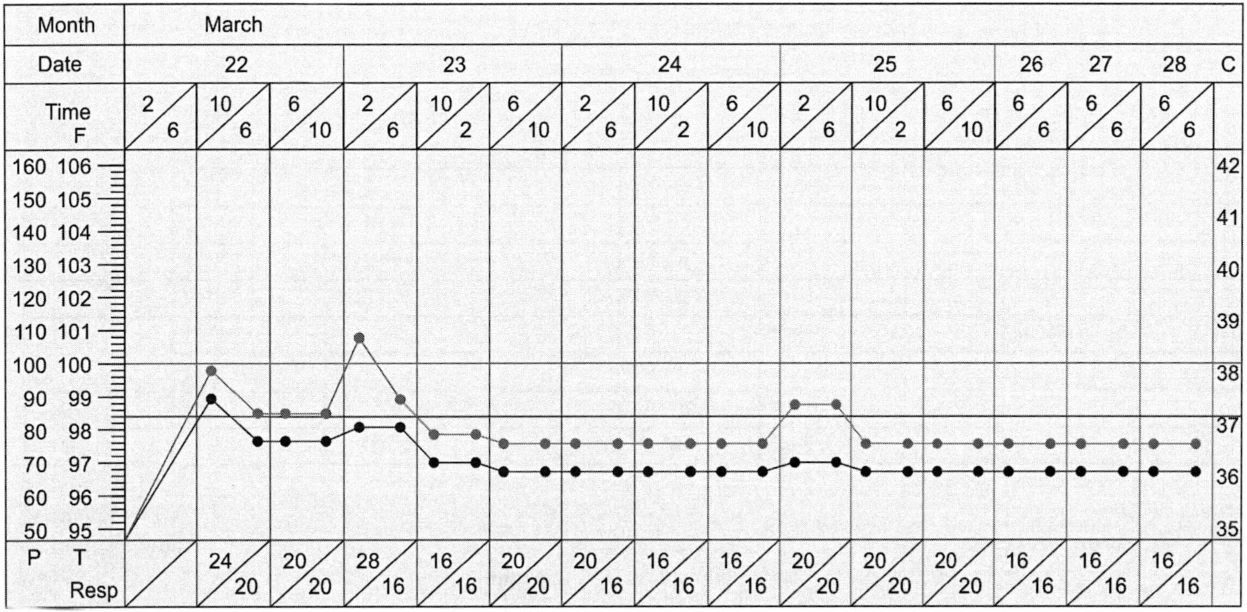

Table 6.1: Intake and output chart

Patient's Name:
Age: 30 years

Ward No. 6
Female Surgical Ward
Bed No. 5

Date	Time	Intake	Amount	Output	Amount
22/3/13	10 am	IV Dextrose 5%	540 mL		
	12 Noon	Juice	200 mL		
	1 pm			Vomit	200 mL
	2 pm	Milk	200 mL		
	4 pm	IV Normal saline	500 mL		
	6 pm	IV Ringer lactate	900 mL		
	10 pm	Milk	200 mL	Urine	400 mL

Table 6.2: Nurses notes

Ward No: 5
Medical Ward

Patient's Name:
Bed No. 4, Age: 45 years
Reg No. 1234

Date	Time	Notes
25/3/13	10 am	Client was admitted with dyspnea, cyanosis, cough with expectorations. Assessment was done. Vital signs checked after giving Fowler's bed and position. O_2 inhalation started. Temperature normal, pulse 84/min, respiration 30/min, BP 120/80 mm of Hg, general condition fair
	12 Noon	Nebulization was given, discontinuing oxygen, sputum mug provided to spit
	1 pm	Food was served. Light diet given
	2 pm	Vital signs checked. They are normal. T98P, T4, R 24/min. Oxygen inhalation discontinued
	4 pm	Oral liquids given—juice 250 mL
	6 pm	Vitals checked. Patient is having 103°F temperature. Cold compress and ice cap given, medicines given as ordered
	8 pm	Temperature came to normal
	9 pm	Light diet given. Oral fluids given
	10 pm	Nebulization given

Vague terms and phrases should not be used. It must be accurate. Avoid use of unnecessary words and irrelevant details. It must be complete containing appropriate and essential information.

Timely entries are essential in ongoing care, e.g. vital signs, medicines, treatment and nursing interventions, admission, discharge, death, etc.

It is to be in logical order, organized notes describing heath problem, assessment intervention and client's response. Records should reflect accountability. Signature holds that nurse is responsible, e.g. for her observations, actions, spelling and use of any institution's accepted abbreviations, symbols and system of markers are used and each one uses the same and avoids misinterpretation.

Methods

- **Problem-oriented medical record:** It has database, problem list, core plan and progress notes
  - **Database:** Information about assessment. History, findings of physical examination, ongoing assessment and laboratory reports
  - **Problem list:** Problems are identified from date and list. Problems are arranged in chronological order filed infront of clients record, date is mentioned against the resolved problem
  - **Nursing care plan:** Care plan is prepared as per problems which includes nursing diagnosis, expected outcome, nursing intervention and evaluation
  - **Progress notes:** Progress of client is monitored and expressed in structured format.
- **SOAP:** S, Subjective data—data collected from patient relatives. O, objective data—observations made, investigation reports, e.g. vital signs, blood sugar, weight signs. A—assessment, interpreting subjective and objective data—nursing diagnosis. P, Plan—plan of nursing care which includes expected outcome and action to be taken
- **Narrative documentation:** Traditional method for recording nursing care, story type recording
- **PIE:** P—Problem, I—Intervention, E—Evaluation
- **Charting by exception:** Standardized statements are on the forms. If it is not in the format, nurse charts what is observed out of ordinary or has occurred.
- **Case management plan and critical pathway:** It is a model of delivering care. It has multidisciplinary approach to document client

care. It has time frame. Unexpected outcomes, if they occur are called as variances.

Common Formats

History: Refer page no. 107
Assessment: Refer page no. 91, 97
Nursing care plan: Refer page no 65, 72.
Nurses notes: Refer page no. 68
Flow sheets: It includes graphic record of temperature (T), pulse (P), respiration (R) and blood pressure (BP), medicines administered, intake output and wound assessment record.
Graphic record: Temperature chart, bar diagram, partogram, growth chart.
Kardex: This system consists of series of cards kept in a portable index file or form. It contains following information. Client's name, age, sex, religion, marital status, admission date, time, ward no, phone no, physician's name, diagnosis, medications, IV fluids daily treatment procedures, vital signs, investigations, allergies, activities permitted, assistance needed and special instructions, if any.
Audit records.

STANDARDIZED CARE PLANS

Care plans are preprinted depending on the standard practice. After assessment, nurse selects the appropriate standard care plan and is kept in client's record. Modification can be made in ink to individualize therapies, care plans are updated regularly.

Discharge summary forms. It has instructions in nutrition and drugs. Rehabilitative techniques. Community resources available, conditions to seek medical care, follow-up.

Methods of obtaining follow-up care, responsibility of family members. Medication instructions.

Computerized documentation—System can be used for supplies, e.g. equipment, drugs, diagnosis tests. Standard formats are developed, software programs allow nurses to enter data quickly. Care plans also can be prepared from data in computer. Computer-based patient care record (CPCR) is comprehensive system that uses many components of data collection.

REPORTS

Reports are timely, accurate and relevant.

Change of shift reports. Nurses give report about clients information to nurses working on next shift when leaving.

It provides continuity of care. It may be given orally in person, during walking planning rounded at each client's bedside. It can also be given in conference room. Review of significant record should be done.

Telephone Reports

Information about client to doctors, laboratory staff, other departments can be given or received on phone. Record the time, information, who was called, to whom information was given.

Transfer Report

It may be given personally or on phone. Name, age, limited diagnosis, progress, current health status, allergies, emergency code status, family support, nursing diagnosis, intervention to be done, special, e.g. equipment needed.

Incident Reports

Any event not consistent with routine health care delivery.

Client fall, needle stick injury, visitors have symptoms of illness, medication errors, accidental omission of therapies, injury or risk.

INSTITUTIONAL CARE PLANS (REFER TO PAGE NO 66)

Kardex: Card Filing System

Provides information regarding nursing care, medications, activity levels, level of self-care, diet, treatments and procedures.

Nursing care plan is inside the card. (Refer to page no 73)

CHAPTER

7

Vital Signs, Body Temperature, Physiology, and Regulation

AIM

Students demonstrate the ability to monitor client's vital signs accurately.

OBJECTIVES

- Students know how to assess client's body temperature, pulse, and blood pressure accurately
- Students learn to take care of thermometers and sphygmomanometer.

VITAL SIGNS, BODY TEMPERATURE, PHYSIOLOGY, AND REGULATION

Body produces and conserves heat. Normally, hypothalamus situated between two cerebral hemispheres controls body temperature. Comfortable set point at which heating system operates is comfortable temperature.

Hypothalamus senses minor changes in temperature. Anterior hypothalamus controls heat loss and posterior controls heat production.

Heat is lost by sweating, vasodilatation, and inhibition of heat production. Posterior thalamus senses body's temperature when lower than the set point and heat conservation mechanisms are instituted. Vasoconstriction reduces flow to skin and extremities. Heat is produced through voluntary muscle contraction and muscle shivering.

Factors Affecting Body Temperature

Age

In newborn, temperature fluctuates as the temperature regulation mechanisms is not well-developed and a sudden change of environment. Extra care is needed to protect from environment. Adequate clothing and avoiding exposure helps in maintaining body temperature between 35.5°C to 37.5°C. Temperature regulation is unstable until children reach puberty. Older adults are sensitive to temperature extremes.

Exercise

Muscle activity requires increased blood supply and energy. Increased metabolism causes increase in heat production and raise temporary body temperature.

Hormone Level

Women have more body temperature fluctuations than men. Menstrual cycle, progesterone level, menopause makes changes in body temperature, increased at time of ovulation, hot flushes in menopause.

Stress

Physical, emotional stress increases body temperature.

Environment

Environmental temperature affects body temperature, infants and old people are more sensitive.

Temperature Alterations

Changes affect the hypothalamus set point in relation to excessive heat production, loss, minimal heat production and loss.

Assessment of Body Temperature

Types of thermometers—glass thermometers (Fig. 7.2), electronic thermometers, disposable thermometers, tympanic thermometers, Swan-Ganz catheter (Table 7.1).

Table 7.1: Types of thermometers used in assessment of body temperature

Chemical dot thermometers contain chemical units which change with specific temperature. It is to be removed from wrapper and placed under the tongue for one minute. Patient can bite down safely onto these thermometers	Infrared rays emitted by tympanic membrane in the ear are sensed with this thermometer. It is accurate measurement of core temperature as the blood supply is same to tympanic membrane and hypothalamus Probe tip has autoscope shape and probe is gently placed in ear canal putting pinna back reading is obtained in 2–3 seconds	Catheter contains thermistor that can be attached to cardiac computer Catheter is in pulmonary artery
Electronic thermometers consists of battery pack with probe attached and disposable probe covers. Reading is taken within 2–60 seconds Different probes or same probe is used for different routes. So, read instructions before use	Glass thermometers • Clinical with elongated bulb • Rectal with round bulb These are cylindrical with mercury inside. Parts – Bulb, Stem, Range of temperature marking is from 35°C to 42°C in centigrade scale and 95°F to 110°F in fahrenheit scale	

Routes of Temperature Monitoring (Table 7.2)

Table 7.2: Different routes of temperature monitoring

Axillary	*Oral*	*Rectal*	*Tympanic*
Wipe dry from bulb to stem. Bring mercury to lowest level by gentle jerk with wrist (snap) Wipe axilla to dry Keep thermometer bulb in axilla and press the arm and ask patient to hold in place keeping hand across the chest. Keep for 3 minutes. Read. Wipe with wet swab from stem to bulb and place in jar	Rinse in cold water dry with swab or clean tissue from bulb to fingers. Read level of mercury, shake down by snapping movement of wrist, moisten in cold water, moisten tips, place thermometer in posterior sublingual area. Ask person to close lips. After 3–4 minutes, wipe off the secretion with tissue from tips to bulb Read and wash	Hold back clothes. Give position, apply lubricant, insert bulb end into anal orifice lifting upper buttock 1 cm in infants, 3–4 cm in adults. Hold in place for 1–2 minute. Remove thermometer. Wipe anal area. Cover person. Read, wash and replace, wash hands (Fig. 7.1)	Probe is gently placed in ear canal putting pinna back Read after three seconds

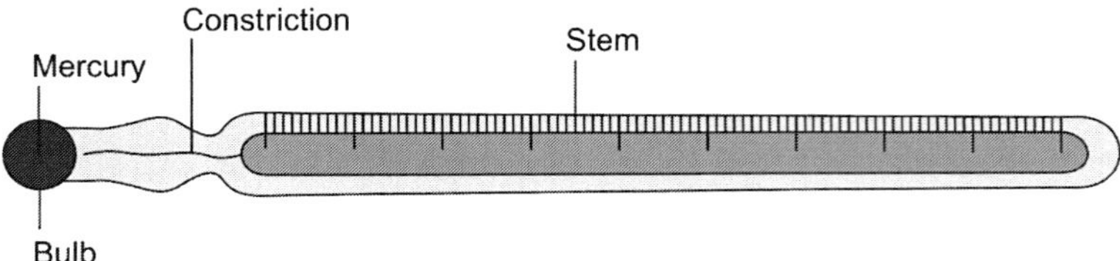

Fig. 7.1: Rectal thermometer

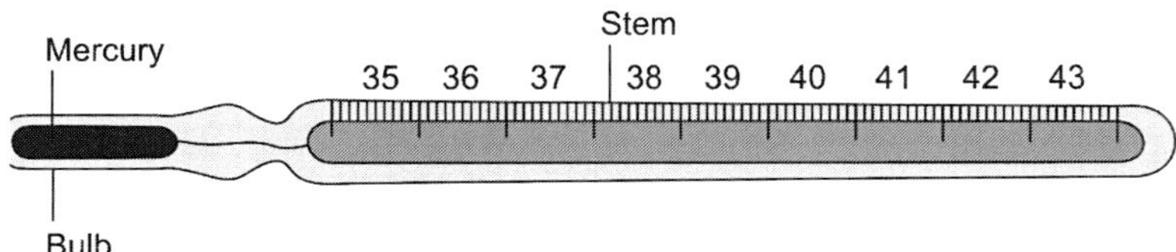

Fig. 7.2: Clinical thermometer

Temperature Alterations

Pyrexia

Cause: Heat loss mechanism is unable to keep pace with excess heat production and result in abnormal rise in body temperature.

Bacteria and viruses cause fever. Pyrogens when enter body act as antigens and stimulate immune system.

Leukocytes are increased to fight against bacteria, harems are released. These factors cause hypothalamus to raise the set point to meet new higher set point.

Febrile: Person having fever.

Afebrile: Person without fever.

Hypothermia: Abnormally low body temperature.

Hyperthermia or hyperpyrexia: Extremely elevated body temperature > 40°C (104°F).

Types:

Low grade fever: > 37. 1°C, < 38. 2°C (99–101°F)

High grade fever: > 38. 2°C (100.4°F)

Relapsing or intermittent fever: Periods of febrile and normal body temperature alternately.

Continuous fever: Continuous ranging from 38.2°C to 40°C without reaching to normal.

Fever of underdetermined origin (FUO)/Pyrexia of unknown origin (PUO)

Management

- Reduce fever
- Maintain optimal nutrition
- Maintain fluid and electrolyte balance
- Promote comfort and rest
- Eliminate cause of fever
- Provide for home management.

Hypothermia

Temperature below normal
Types:
Mild: 35°C–32°C
Moderate: 32°C–26°C
Deep: below 26°C
Causes: Exposure to cold, wet, windy climate. Accidental immersion in cold water. Sking, mountain climbing. Homeless people, infants, children with immature regulatory centers alcohol.

Management

- Rewarming
- Placing in warm, dry environment
- Extra blankets
- Careful monitoring
- Fluid and electrolyte replacement
- Antibiotics.

HEAT STROKE

It is a severe life-threatening condition resulting from prolonged exposure to heat.

It is profound disturbance of body's heat regulating mechanism caused by prolonged exposure to excessive heat from sun. Person over 40 and those in poor health are most susceptible to it. First aid includes moving a client to cooler environment, remove clothes, placing cool wet towels over skin and use of fans to increase heat loss. IV fluids, irrigation of stomach and cooler with cool water. Use of hypothermia blankets.

Monitor rectal temperature. Ice cap over head. Cold pack, if temperature above 104°F (40°C).

COLD AND HOT APPLICATIONS

Applying cold or heat to the body.

Purposes

- To reduce or increase body temperature
- To reduce edema, inflammation
- To provide warm environment
- To stop hemorrhage
- To accelerate healing process
- To relieve pain
- To stimulate nerves for muscle activity
- To reduce hematoma
- To dilate or constrict blood vessels.

LOCAL APPLICATION

Local: Hot—hot water bag, hot compress, electric pad, sister kenny's pack.
Cold: Ice cap, ice collar, cold compress, sucking ice cubes.
Warm: Sitz bath, irrigation, foot bath, douche.
General: Cold—cold pack, ice water enema, cold sponge, tepid sponge.

Cold or hot applications constrict or dilate blood vessels to help in reduction or increase in blood supply to effect on removal of toxins, accelerate sweating, stimulation of nerve endings and relief of discomfort.

Filling of Hot Water Bag

Hot water bag (Fig. 7.3) is rubber article specially prepared with thick rubber to tolerate 160°F or more temperature. It is dried well before keeping in cupboard and air is introduced to keep two surfaces apart.

When filled and applied over patient's body surface is filled with water 120°F to 160°F temperature and air is removed before cork is applied.

Equipment Required

- Hot water bag (Fig. 7.3)
- Clean cloth
- Hot water in jug, cold water

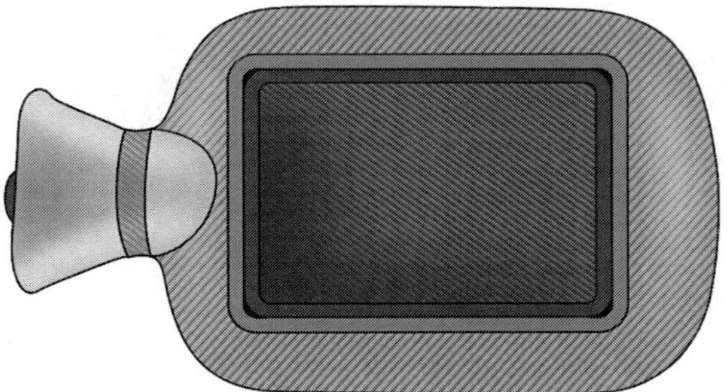

Fig. 7.3: Hot water bag

- Point measure
- Funnel.

Procedure

- Measure capacity of bag with cold water
- Mix hot and cold water to 140°F or 60°C in point measure for unconscious patient only 120°F or 49°C
- Open cork and pour hot water of 60°C temperature by funnel into bag slowly. As the water enters, air will come out slowly
- While pouring, rest the hot water bag on table and pour the water
- Holding on table press against body, still water is seen near the neck of bag. Put cork and close tightly confirming air is out. Hold upside down
- Wipe with clean cloth
- Put cover and wrap in towel or cloth
- Take to the patient
- Explain the procedure, if patient is conscious
- Apply over body surface where needed.

Filled hot water bag may be applied over lower abdomen for full bladder, extremities, chest for warmth and pain relief, at foot, or kept in bed near body, over back for local warmth. To keep bed warm in admission bed, operation bed before patient is received.

Filling and Applying Ice Cap

Equipment

Tray containing ice cap (Fig. 7.4) with cover, ice cubes in bowl, bowl with water, salt, tablespoon and piece of cloth.

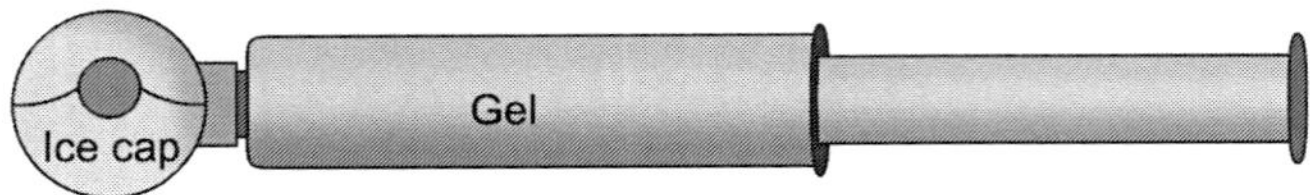

Fig. 7.4: Prefilled ice pack

Procedure

Check ice cap for leakage. Smoothen edges of ice cubes by dipping in water and place inside the ice cap after opening the cork. Fill 2/3rd, add one teaspoon salt. Remove air and place cork. Wipe from outside with cloth and apply cover.

Apply to the body areas of patient like head, abdomen, wound, injection site, etc. Keep till ice melts. Refill, if needed. Clean and dry and replace by filling air. Wash hands. Document the intervention on nurses notes.

Medical Fomentation

It is an application of heat to the inflamed, painful part of the body. It is a clean technique.

Equipment

- A tray containing medium-sized bowl, ringer, lint pieces
- 5×3 size cotton pad, piece of plastic, bandage, boiling water in point measure
- Mackintosh and towel.

Procedure

- Check the order
- Screen the patient
- Explain the procedure to patient. Switch off fan, place mackintosh and towel under the part to be fomented
- Adjust the tray at safe place as it has boiling water
- Spread ringer on bowl. Place folded lint piece in bowl
- Pour boiling water over lint piece
- Ring out the water with sticks attached to ringer
- Place lint piece on inflamed part, place plasic piece, cotton pad and bandage

- Repeat the procedure as ordered
- Observe the area before next application
- If not tolerated the heat, apply vaseline and keep open.

Surgical Fomentation

It is a application of heat to the wound. It is sterile procedure and aseptic technique is to be used.

Equipment

Lint pieces boiled in water, bowl of boiling water, two dissecting forceps, sterile cotton pad and bandage, gloves, mackintosh, and towel.

Procedure

Wash hands. Expose wound. Observe the wound. Place mackintosh and towel under the part. Wash hands and wear gloves. Wring out lint piece with dissecting forceps and place on the wound. Apply cotton pad and bandage. Repeat the procedure as ordered. Wash hands. Remove gloves. Remove mackintosh and towel. Wash articles. Send forceps for autoclaving.

Cold Compress

Folded piece of cloth dipped in ice water are kept on forehead or in groins, axilla to reduce body temperature.

Equipment

Small tray with ice water in bowl, ice, two pieces of lint cloth, mackintosh small and towel.

Procedure

Carry the tray to patient after identifying the patient. Explain the procedure to patient, if conscious. Keep mackintosh under the body part where compress is applied, eg. forehead, swollen area. Put ice cubes in water bowl. Fold lint piece and dip into water. Hold one end of cloth in left hand and remove water by pressing and withdrawing cloth with index and middle finger of right hand. Place on forehead from lateral to medial side. Change cloth after it dries by wetting it again and replacing. Carry out procedure for 15–20 minutes. Teach the procedure to relative. After procedure is complete check the patient's body temperature. Replace the articles after washing with soap and water and drying.

Tepid Sponge

Sponging body with tap water to reduce temperature in fever 102°–103° F.

Equipment

Basin, jug with tap water, sponge cloths five, mackintosh, towel, bedsheet, cold compress, and ice cap.

Procedure

Check the patient's body temperature. Provide privacy. Explain the procedure to patient. Spread long mackintosh over bed underneath. Place hot water bag at feet. Fan fold top linen and place near foot end. Cover the patient with single sheet and remove clothes. Spread bath towel over chest and other on pelvic region. Pour tap water into basin and wet five sponge bags. Take first sponge bag, wipe face and put it on the edge of the basin. Take a second sponge bag, wipe distal arm starting from acromian process proceeding laterally to fingers, and reach axilla. Place sponge bag in axilla. Take a third sponge bag and wipe proximal arm in the same way, and place sponge bag in axilla. Wipe abdomen and back with first sponge bag which was left on edge of the basin. For legs, start from thigh, proceed laterally to feet and medially to groin and keep cloth in groin. Wipe face and neck again. Take sponge cloth from axilla, dip and squeeze and repeat procedure for proximal and distal hand. Check body temperature every 15 minutes, observe for chills, cyanosis and check pulse. Continue procedure for 15–20 minutes. Remove sponge cloths, dry the patient. Remove mackintosh, cover with sheet. Remove towels. Change patient's clothes. Make patient comfortable. Clean and replace articles.

Cold Sponge

The procedure is same as tepid sponge, but the water temperature is 20–30° C.

Cold Pack

This is used in management of patients with heat stroke, when patient's body temperature is 40°C or above 104°F.

Equipment

Ice cap, cold compress, large mackintosh, bedsheet, basin with ice water, thermometer.

Procedure

Spread full mackintosh over bed. Explain the procedure to patient. Screen the bed. Cover him with single sheet and remove clothes. Dip bedsheet in cold water and wring out. Keep ice cap on head and cold compress on forehead. Turn the patient to one side. Place wet bedsheet along the side in length. Spread sheet and roll the patient over it. Wrap sheet around body and keep for 10–15 minutes. Remove wet sheet, mackintosh and wipe dry. Take rectal temperature. If not reduced, repeat the procedure.

PULSE: PHYSIOLOGY, REGULATIONS, CHARACTERISTICS

The local rhythmic expansion of an artery which can be felt with the finger, corresponding to each contraction of left ventricle of the heart. It can be felt in any artery, sufficiently near the surface of the body which passes over a bone and the normal adult rate, if 72 beats/min. In children it is more rapid varying from 130 in infants to 80 in older children.

Electrical impulse originating from sinoatrial (SA) node travel through heart muscle to stimulate cardiac contraction with each contraction 70 mL of blood is pushed into aorta (stroke volume) and walls of the aorta distends creating pulse wave that travels rapidly towards distal end of the arteries. Pulse wave moves 15 times faster through aorta and 100 times faster through small arteries.

Pulse is the palpable bounding of the blood flow in the peripheral artery. Cardiac output is the volume of blood pumped by the heart during each minute. 70 × 70 = 4900 mL. Mechanical, neural and chemical factors regulate the strength of heart contractions and stroke volume.

Characteristics

Rate

Baseline measurement is done as there are fluctuations in rate with change of position like sitting, standing, lying down. Rate is number of beats per minute. Pulse rate varies depending on age, level of activity, exercise, fever, pain, anxiety, medications and hemorrhage.

Rhythm

Interval between two pulse beats. Equal interval is present in normal pulse, late beat, missed beat in diabetes, dysrhythmia.

Strength

Amplitude of pulse reflects volume of blood ejected. It is same at each heart beat. Description may be strong, weak, thready, bounding depending on the strength or volume.

Equality

On both sides should be equal.

Factors Affecting Pulse

Emotion

Pulse is increased or decreased when emotionally disturbed, e.g. fear, anger.

Exercise

Muscle activity increases metabolic rate, cardiac output and increase in pulse due to increase peripheral blood.

Position

When sitting, pulse is normal and increased on standing. Normal in resting and lying down position.

Race

Black races like Negro pulse rate is higher than white.

Sex

Females have faster pulse rate than males.

Age

High pulse rate in newborn, gradually decreases till adulthood.

Drugs

Cardiac stimulants increases pulse rate. Digoxin decreases pulse rate.

Condition of Blood Vessels

When lumen of arteries is decreased, pulse increases in arteriosclerosis.

Blood Volume

Pulse is directly proportional to the volume of blood circulating in the body.

Hormone

Thyroxine increases pulse rate.

High Altitude

Pulse increases at high altitude.

Sites

Radial, apical, temporal, carotid, brachial, femoral, popliteal, dorsalis pedis, posterior tibial (Fig. 7.5).

Rate

Number of beats per minute.

Normal: Neonates and infants 120/mm

2 years	110/mm
4 years – 6 years	100/mm
8 years – 12 years	90/mm
12 years – 14 years	80 + 90/mm
16 years – 18 years	70 + 80/mm
Well-conditioned	50 + 60/mm
Athlete	
Adult	60–100/mm
Aging	60 + 100/mm

Tachycardia: 100 beats/mm in adults.

Causes: Exercise, fever, hypoxemia, cardiac problems, hypertension, pain, anger, fear, anxiety.

Bradycardia: 60 beats/mm.

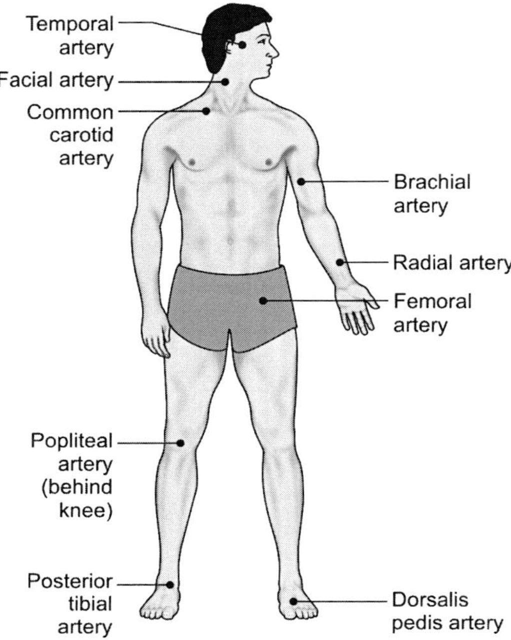

Fig. 7.5: Main pulse point

Causes: Digitalis, vomiting, suctioning, cardiac conduction problems, raised intracranial pressure.

Rhythm

It is to be regular in normal condition, there may be many irregularities. Sinus arrhythmia, premature beats, totally irregular.

Pulse Deficit

Exists when apical pulse is more than radial pulse. It indicates inefficient contraction of the ventricle.

Pulse Force

If stroke volume decreases—weak thready pulse; if increases bounding pulse also in heart block, anemia, hepatic failure, aortic insufficiency.

Pulse Oximeter

It is photoelectric device that measures oxygen saturation of the arterial blood at peripheral sites.

- Probe is attached to a finger, toe, earlobe, or bridge of the nose
- It contains sensors which measure amount of HB (oxygenated or reduced)
- Electronic black box interprets the ratio of it
- Percentage (%) is displayed on visual screen.

Normal oxygen saturation is 97–99%, below 94% respiratory compromise, below 91% needs oxygen therapy and intubations.

Hemodynamic pressure monitoring

- **Swan-Ganz catheter:** It is double lumen catheter threaded into thoracic vein through right side of the heart. End is in pulmonary artery. It indicates amount of circulating blood volume, pumping efficiency of the heart and vascular tone. Pressure increases with cardiac failure
- **Central venous pressure (CVP):** Pressure in the right atrium of the heart through Swan-Ganz catheter, CVP catheter. It is threaded through view into superior or inferior vena cava.

RESPIRATION: PHYSIOLOGY, REGULATIONS

Tissues of the body utilize the oxygen for metabolic process and give up carbon dioxide. Respiratory system provides oxygen from the atmosphere to the tissues and takes out carbon dioxide from the tissues and discharge it into atmosphere (Fig. 7.6). Lungs expand, inflate and atmospheric air enters in. Oxygen is taken by blood and circulated to tissues. Carbon dioxide is diffused out into blood.

External Respiration

External respiration consists of inspiration, expiration and pause.

Internal Respiration (Fig. 7.7)

Hemoglobin in blood releases oxygen (O_2) to cells and cells release carbon dioxide (CO_2).

Respiration is automatic and involuntary, but it can be controlled voluntarily. Normally respiratory patterns changes according to cellular demands.

Respiratory center in brainstem controls the rate, rhythm and depth of respiration. Reflexes, chemicals and control by higher centers regulate

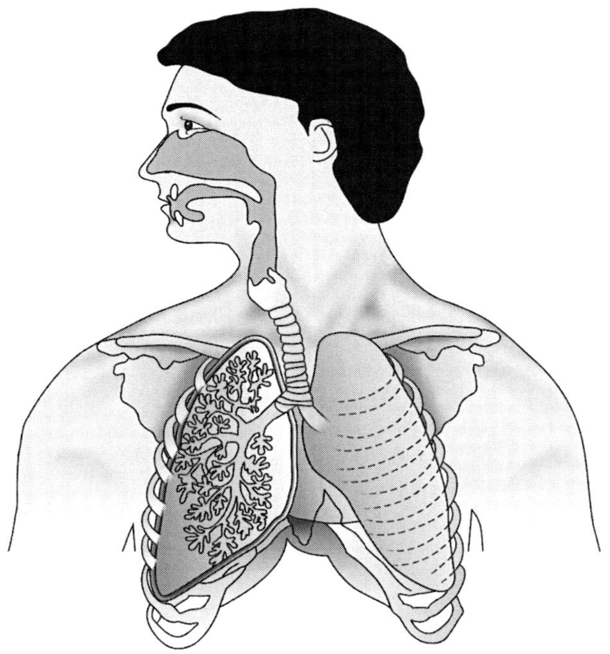

Fig. 7.6: Respiratory system

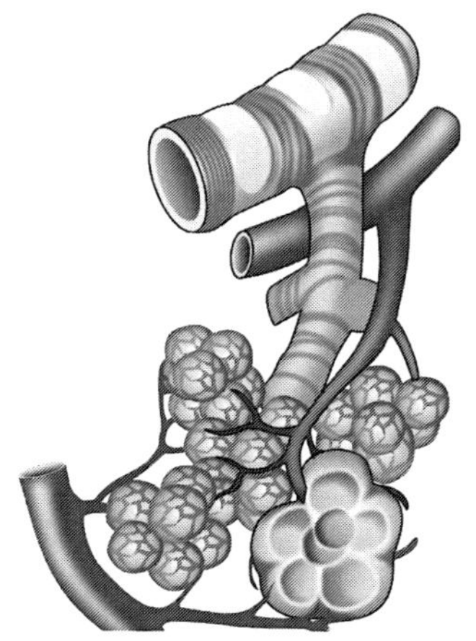

Fig. 7.7: Internal respiratory system

respirations. Reflexes—Hering-Breuer reflex—sensors present in bronchioles, receptors in capillaries, reflexes from muscles, joints, lung irritant receptors, peripheral chemoreceptors, baroreceptors in arteries control respirations.

Chemicals

Carbon dioxide tension of arterial blood $PaCO_2$ is influencing factor of control of respiration. CO_2 acts 70% on central chemoreceptors and 30% on peripheral chemoreceptors. Oxygen fall in arterial blood PaO_2 causes stimulation of respiration. Fall of blood pH in acidosis causes hyperventilation and in alkalosis hypoventilation.

Mechanics

During inspiration, chest wall expands and intrapulmonary pressure is reduced, air from atmosphere enters lungs. During expiration, chest wall and lungs shrink, intrapulmonary pressure rises, air is forced out of lungs. Expansion and shrinkage of thoracic wall and lungs is called as ventilation. Muscles of inspiration contract and cause expansion of thoracic cage in transverse, vertical and anteroposterior diameter. Parietal pleura attached to inner side of chest wall and visceral pleura moves and lungs expand. Expansion of lungs causes dilatation of airway tube and alveoli and pressure falls. External air enters through nose, pharynx, trachea, bronchi, and bronchioles into alveoli. Muscles of respiration relax resulting in elastic recoil of lungs and intrapulmonary pressure rises and expired air leaves lungs. Thus, the mechanism of respiration consists of inspiration, expiration, pause. Diaphragm and intercostal muscles are muscles of respiration.

Characteristics

It is automatic, involuntary, regular, rhythmic, 12–16 times per minute in adults, 20–40 per minute in children. Volume of air inspired and expired is 500 mL in each respiration. It can be increased voluntarily.

Factors Affecting Respiration

Sudden stress, exercise, environment, change in altitude, adjustment made for singing, laughing, speaking, crying, swallowing, defecating, etc.

Assessment

Ask the patient to be comfortable in lying down position. If difficulty in lying down position give comfortable Fowler's position. Observe the movements of the chest. One inspiration is, inspiration + expiration. Count inspirations for one minute. Observe for any abnormality, depth of respiration.

Alterations

Normal respiration is effortless, automatic, regular, and even.
Orthopnea: Inability to breathe on lying down.
Dyspnea: Difficult, labored or painful breathing.
Stertorous: Noisy—due to secretions in respiratory tract.
Stridor: Harsh, inspiratory crowing sound—due to laryngeal obstruction.
Wheezing: High pitched, musical whistling sound due to partial obstruction in bronchi and bronchioles.
Sighing: Deep inspiration followed by prolonged expiration:
Rate and depth:
Upto 1 year of age - 30–40/min
1–4 years - 20–30/min
4–10 years - 20–26/min
12–18 years - 12–20/min
Adult - 10–20/min

Normal Respiratory Movements

Inspiration

It is an active process. Respiratory center sends nerve impulses along the phrenic nerve causing diaphragm to contract. Abdominal organs move forward, increase length of chest cavity to move air into lungs.

Diaphragm moves 1 cm and ribs retract upward 1.2–2. 5 cm; person inhales about 500 mL of air (tidal volume).

Expiration

It is a passive process, diaphragm relaxes and abdominal organs return to their original position. Lung and chest wall returns to relaxed position.

Eupnea is normal rate and depth of respiration during quiet breathing chest wall gently rises and falls.

In difficult breathing, contraction of neck muscles, intercostal muscles is present and are visible and not in quite breathing. Indrawing of sternum is a serious sign in pneumonia.

Comfortable position like Fowler's position, cardiac position, extra support helps in breathing easily.

Cleaning of crust in nostrils, pharynx suctioning, endotracheal suction helps to remove obstruction from upper respiratory tract.

Preventing falling back of tongue by turning head to one side or putting airway, ¾ prone position will help in breathing in semiconscious and unconscious patients.

Oxygen therapy in cyanosis will help to bring breathing to normal. Deep breathing exercises preoperatively and after operation will help to maintain normal respiration. Relief from axiety, pain will help in maintaining normal respiration, administering medications, inhalation will help patient to get relief from difficulty in breathing.

Helping the patient to cough out expectorations, tapping the chest and back will help in relieving chest congestion.

Application of heat to chest and back or wrapping warm shawl or blanket, jacket, warm clothes will help to improve breathing in cold weather.

Depth in inhaled and exaled volume of air during each respiration. Tidal volume is about 500–800 mL. Spirometer is used to measure tidal volume.

Tachypnea : 24 breaths/min
Bradypnea : 10 breaths/min
Hypoventilation : Reduced amount of air reaching to alveoli.
Apnea : Cessation of breathing.

Hyperventilation

Increase in rate and depth of respiration, kussmaul's breathing in diabetic acidosis, causes low levels of pCO_2 and pH>7.45.

Biot's Respiration

Irregular breathing pattern, 10 seconds to 1 minute duration same depth. $PaCO_2$ is partial pressure of CO_2 in arterial blood and is reflection of the depth of pulmonary ventilation.

Normal range is 35–45 mm of Hg.

<35 mm of Hg — Hypoventilation
>45 mm of Hg — Hyperventilation

PaO_2 is partial pressure of oxygen in arterial blood. Normal range is 80–100 mm Hg.
< 60 mm of Hg—anaerobic—lactic—metabolic acidosis
Hypoxemia—hyperventilation—respiratory alkalosis
Arterial blood gas analysis is best way to evaluate acid-base balance.
pH measures hydrogen ion (H^+) concentration in body fluids.
Blood—Normal pH value is 7.35–7.45.
<7.35 acidic, < 7.45 alkaline
O_2 saturation—Point at which Hb is saturated with oxygen.
Normal value is 95–99%.
Bicarbonate (HCO_3) is major renal component of acid-base balance. Excreted and reproduced as per need by kidneys to maintain acid-base balance. Normal range is 22–26 mg/L.

>24 mg/L	-	metabolic acidosis
<28 mg/L	-	" alkalosis"
Respiratory acidosis	-	increased $PaCO_2$ "H_2CO_3 decreased pH".

BLOOD PRESSURE

Definition

It is the lateral pressure exerted by blood on the walls of the vessels in which it contains. Force exerted by blood on the walls of blood vessels.
Systolic pressure: Pressure exerted during contraction of left ventricle of the heart.
Diastolic pressure: Pressure exerted during relaxation of ventricles of the heart.
Pulse pressure: The difference between systolic and diastolic pressure.
Regulation: Neural control and local control—chemical and autoregulatory.
Neural control: Medulla contains vasomotor center.

Sympathetic fibers are vasoconstrictors and parasympathetic vasodilators. Sympathetic stimulation leads to vasoconstriction in skin and splanchnic blood vessels. Vasomotor center is influenced by sinoaortic baroreceptors, carotid aortic chemoreceptors, cardiopulmonary reflexes, acute pain, reduced oxygen concentration and composition of arterial blood affects vasomotor center.

Regulation of blood pressure means mechanism by which the blood pressure homeostasis is maintained. BP = Cardiac output × peripheral resistance.

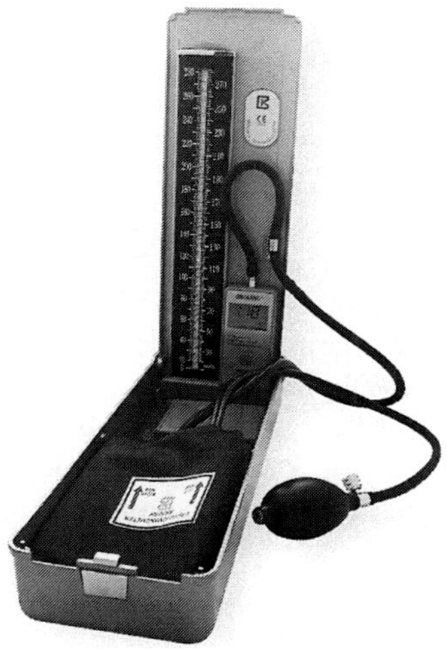

Fig. 7.8: Sphygmomanometer

Factors Affecting Blood Pressure

- Cardiac output
- Peripheral vascular resistance
- Elasticity of the arteries
- Blood volume
- Blood viscosity
- Age, sex/gender, weight, race, climate, diet, circadian rhythm, exercise, stress, position.

Instrument used to measure blood pressure is sphygmomanometer (Fig. 7.8), mercury manometer. It consists of:

- Pressure manometer
- Compression cuff
- Calibrated glass column.

Aneroid manometer: It consist of:

- Metal below inside gauge
- Compression cuff
- Calibrated dial.

They are portable and easy to read.

Techniques

Auscultatory

- Placing cuff on brachial artery
- Inflating cuff
- Placing stethoscope in cubital fossa to listen korotkoff sounds
- Releasing cuff and reducing pressure
- As the pressure is reduced, stopped blood flow starts
- Ist reappearance of clear tapping sounds is systolic pressure. Note the reading, two consecutive beats (Phase I)
- Phase II and III are subtle sounds and not heard
- Phase IV and V, phase IV is muffling sound phase and V is the point at which tapping sound disappears completely. Reading at this point is diastolic pressure.

Palpatory Method

Fingers are used instead of stethoscope to palpate radial artery. Systolic pressure can be noted in this method.

Cardiac Monitor

- Electrodes are posted on the chest
- Connected to oscilloscope or screen
- Electrical impulses are transmitted through electrodes.

Doppler

- Place drop of coupling gel on the transducer
- Place transducer on arterial pulse
- Hold the probe on the skin tilted 40° angle
- Put the device on, listen to the sound.

CHAPTER

8

Health Assessment

AIM

Students are able to make health assessment.

OBJECTIVES

- Students are able to collect data
- Students perform physical examination.

HEALTH ASSESSMENT

Concept and Importance of Assessment

Assessment is the deliberate and systematic collection of data to determine a client's current and past health status, tensional status and coping patterns. It has two steps:

1. Collection and verifications of data from primary source, the patient and secondary sources family, health professional and medical records.
2. Analysis of data to develop nursing diagnosis and care plan.

Purpose

- To establish database about the client's perceived needs, health problems and responses to these problems
- To reveal related experiences, health practice goals, values and expectations about health system. Data collection includes subjective and objective data from or about a patient.

Subjective data: It is patient's perception about his/her health problems. Only patient can provide this information, e.g. pain, fear, anxiety, stress. These problems may be manifested physiologically and nurse can identify them with observation through objective data collection.

Objective data: It is observations or measurements made by the data collector. Assessment of wound—size depth, type, descriptions of behaviors, measurement of height, weight, temperature, pulse, respiration, blood pressure.

Source of data: Patient family, significant others, health professionals, records. Objective data are obtained from physical examination, laboratory reports. Patient can provide data regarding healthcare needs, lifestyle, present and past illness, perceptions of symptoms, change in activities of daily living.

Family and significant others can be primary source of information about infants, children, critically ill patients and mentally challenged, disoriented or unconscious patients. They can give information about illness, medications, allergen, etc. As secondary source of information, they can confirm findings provided by patients. Family and friends can make observations regarding client needs. Health team member can give information about patients regarding medications treatments, response, progress, prognosis, etc. Data in the record are baseline information about patient's response to illness, laboratory reports, medical history, proposed treatment, etc.

BIOGRAPHICAL INFORMATION

- Client's age, address, occupation, working status, marital status, children, source of health care, types of insurance to be included
- **Reasons for seeking health care:** Clients's response, perception for seeking health care
- **Expectations:** Expectations regarding information, about treatment, quality care, outcome of treatment, cleanliness of environment and relief
- **Present illness:** Nature and onset of illness, sudden or gradual, always present or come and go, duration, location, intensity and quality of each symptom. If any action, symptoms precipitate
- **Health history:** If hospitalized before or undergone any surgery, medicines taken, allergies, habits, lifestyle pattern, sleep pattern, nutrition.
- **Family history:** Information about immediate and blood relatives to find out risk for illness of genetic or familial nature and supports relationship

- **Environmental history:** Provides data about client's home and working environment
- **Psychosocial history:** Support system—spouse children, other family members, close friends, ways of coping with stress, recent loss and grief
- **Spiritual health:** Beliefs about life, source of guidance, faith, rituals and religious practices.

BASIC SKILLS IN INTERVIEWING PATIENTS

Interview: Interview is a pattern of communication initiated for specific purpose and focused on a specific content area.

Purpose

- To obtain nursing health history
- To identify health needs and risk factors
- To determine changes in level of wellness and pattern of living
- To obtain information about client's health, lifestyle, support system, patterns of illness, strengths and limitations and resources
- To establish therapeutic relationship with client.

Information obtained from interview is subjective and is to be validated by objective data.

It initiates nurse-client relationship which helps in sharing information and nurse is able to express level of caring for the client.

In emergency situations, nurse asks questions only related to physical status of client.

Chronic illness or routine follow-up interview may focus on past and present illness, resources, daily activities, etc.

Use open-ended questions to obtain response of more than one or two wards. Client describes health status. Nurse maintains good eye contact and listening skills. Back channeling includes active listening technique such as saying, *uh, huh, yes, alright.* Nurse may ask probing questions to get information. For example, what else is bothering you? Is there any thing which you want to tell me ? Problem-seeking interview will keep to describe and identify the client's specific problems. Asking closed-ended questions will limit the client's answers to yes or no.

Phases of Interview

- Orientation
- Working
- Termination.

Nurse collects data and creates an environment conducive to interview. Time schedule should be without interruption by health personnel, visitors. Provide comfortable and relaxed environment.

Orientation

Before beginning, nurse views purpose of interview, type of data to be collected and method most appropriate for conducting interview. Establish nurse-client relationship. Nurse consciously communicates a sense of trust and confidentiality to client.

Nurse opens an interview by explaining purpose of interview and the type of questions would be asked.

Working

Nurse asks questions to form a database to develop care plan.

Termination

Inform client that interview is coming to an end, e.g. by saying there are two more questions or we will finish within 5 minutes. Patient may ask final question before interview ends.

HISTORY

Baseline data	:	
Name	:	
Age	:	
Religion	:	
Sex	:	
Date of admission	:	
Time of admission	:	
OPD No.	:	
IPD No.	:	
Diagnosis	:	
Address	:	
Personal history	:	

Contd...

Contd...

Past Medical history :

Present Medical history :

Nutritional history :

Family history :

1. Type of family :

2. Number of members :

Key:

Blue: Male :

Yellow: Female :

Red: Dead :

S. No.	*Name*	*Age*	*Sex*	*Relation*	*Education*	*Health*
1.	Prakash	18 year	M	Son	ISc	Good
2.	Manisha	10 year	F	Daughter	5th	Good

Environmental history :

Socioeconomic history :

Investigations done: :

S. No.	*Investigation*	*Normal value*	*Result*	*Remark*
1.	Blood sugar	80–120 mg/100 mL	180 mg	High

Medication: :

S. No.	*Name of the medicine*	*Dose*	*Route*	*Action*	*Nurses responsibility*
1.	Tab Lasix	0.25 mg	Oral	Diuretic	1. Give at day time 2. Check weight

PHYSICAL EXAMINATION

Objectives

- To collect baseline data about the client's health status
- To supplement, confirm, refute data obtained in the history
- To confirm and identify nursing diagnosis
- To make clinical judgment about a client's changing health status and management
- To evaluate physiological outcomes of the care.

Approaches of Physical Examination

- Head-to-toe approach
- Body system approach

- Functional health pattern approach
- Human response pattern approach
- Problem-solving approach.

Methods

Inspection: Observation With Eyes

In good lighting, comfortable position, exposing body parts, inspect for size, shape, color, symmetry, abnormalities and pay attention to details.

General Observation

Gait, posture, body built, feet dangling, limping, contour of shoulders, level of scapula and iliac crest.

Palpation

Use of hands to touch body parts. It is sensitive assessment.

Skin

Temperature, moisture, texture, turgor, tenderness and thickness.

Abdominal Organs

Light palpation and deep palpation 1 cm deep and 2–4 cm deep, respectively.

Palpation

- 1 cm deep and 2–4 cm deep, warm hands and gentle approach
- Nails to be kept short
- Palpate gently, slowly and deliberately using pads of fingertips.

Percussion

Tapping the body with the fingertips to produce abrasion that travels through body tissues. Character of sound determines location, size, density of underlying structure. Abnormal sound suggests fluid, air within organ or body cavity.

Auscultation

Listening to body organs to detect variations from normal. Sounds from cardiovascular system (CVS), respiratory system, gastrointestinal system

(GI). Stethoscope is used. 5 parts of stethoscope—ear pieces, binoculars, tubings, bell chest piece and diaphragm chest piece. It is placed on skin. Bell chest piece—low-pitched sounds, e.g. bowels and lungs. Diaphragm chest piece—vascular and heart.

Learn to recognize frequency, loudness, quality and duration. Peristalsis is heard all over four quadrants of abdomen as intermittent tinkling sound.

Heart Sounds

Point of maximal impulse (PMI) or apical impulse.

Palpate sternal notch, angle of Louis below suprasternal notch between sternal body and manubrium to second costal space by moving down to left side of sternum to fifth intercostal space and laterally to midclavicular line.

- Heart sounds—(S1) high-pitched, dull
  - Lubb
  - Dupp (S2)
- Fetal heart sounds in pregnant woman.

Equipment

- Cotton applicators
- Cytobrush
- Disposable pad
- Drapes
- Eye chart
- Flash light, spot light
- Forms
- Gloves
- Gown for client
- Ophthalmoscope
- Proctoscope
- Papanicolaou smear slides
- Paper towels
- Percussion hammer
- Ruler
- HT scale
- Specimen bottles, slides
- Sphygmomanometer
- Stethoscope
- Swab sponge forceps
- Tape measures
- Thermometer

- Tissues
- Tongue depressor
- Tuning fork
- Vaginal speculum
- Water-soluble lubricant
- Wrist watch with second hand or digital display.

Preparation of Patient/Client

- Physical comfort to be observed
- Ask him to go for toilet, if needed
- Collect specimen, if ordered
- Explain proper method of collection of specimen
- Give hospital clothes
- Provide privacy and time
- Make patient sit or lie down covering with one sheet up to lap
- Keep warm, eliminate drafts
- Give blanket, if cold. Control room temperature, if possible. Ask him, if he is comfortable.

Positioning

General examination: Sitting, supine, dorsal recumbent, prone, left or right lateral.
Special examination: Knee chest, lateral recumbent, lithotomy.

Observations

General appearance and behavior, gender, race, age, signs of distress, body type, posture, gait, body movements, hygiene and grooming, dress, body odor, affect and mood, speech, client abuse, substance abuse.
Height and weight: Same time of the day, same scale and clothes.
Integument: Skin, nails, hair, scalp.
Skin: Oxygenation, circulation, nutrition, local tissue damage, hydration, lesions, edema, melanoma, erythema, jaundice, induration, moisture, temperature, texture, turgor, vascularity, oxygenation (pallor, cyanosis).

Pricks of IM, IV injections, dullness, dryness, crusting, flaking, scaling.
Temperature: By touching with dorsum of hand for impaired circulation and petechial, pinpointed pimple (blue pimple).
Turgor: Grasp fold of skin on back of the forearm or sternal area with fingertips and release.

Edema: Trauma and venous return impairment, stretched and shiny skin, identification of edematous area (pitting edema).

Head-to-Toe Approach (Table 8.1 and 8.2)

Hair and scalp: Hair, integrity of scalp, infection, infestation.
Alopecia: Baldness.
Nails: Condition reflects general health, nutrition, occupation.
Parts: Nail plate and Nail bed.
Nail bed: Color, thickness, shape, texture of nail, condition of surrounding tissue.

Normally transparent, smooth, convex, and surrounding smooth cuticles without inflammation.

Table 8.1: Basics of head-to-toe assessment

	Symptoms
Hand	
Red or brown linear streaks in nail bed	Trauma, cirrhosis of liver, diabetes, hypertension
Splinter	
clubbing	Change in angle of nail base
Beau's lines	Transverse lines
Paronychia	Inflammation of skin at the nail base
Koilonychia	Spoon nails, concave curves
Head	
Eyes	Visual acuity, visual fields, external eye structures, eyebrows, eyelids, ptosis, ectropion or entropion, redness, blink reflex, lacrimal apparatus, conjunctiva and sclera, bulbar and palpebral, conjunctiva, pallor
Pupils and iris	Size, shape, equality, accommodation, reaction to light pupil size change from 3–7 mm
Pinpoint	Opium toxication, internal eye structures seen though ophthalmoscope
Ears	External ear pain, itching, discharge middle ear, autoscope, hearing
Nose and sinuses	Shape, size, color, deformity, inflammation, excoriation, polyps, palpate frontal and maxillary sinuses
Mouth and pharynx	Lip color, texture, hydration, contour and lesions

Contd...

Contd...

Mucosa	Color, hydration, texture, ulcer, abrasion, cyst
Leukoplakia	Precancerous lesion
Gums and teeth	Gingivitis, gums or gingival color, edema, retraction, bleeding, lesions, denture discomfort, tongue and floor of mouth
Tongue and floor of mouth	
Tongue	Color, size, position, texture, movements, coating or lesions, dull red, moist, slightly rough on top, smooth on lateral margins with free movement, see under the tongue for color, cyst, swelling, lesion. Ventral surface is pink and smooth with large veins and frenulum folds
Mouth floor	Hardness, ulcerations
Palate	Color, shape, texture, extra bony prominences or defects, bony growth, exostosis
Pharynx	Infection, inflammation, lesions
Neck	Muscles, lymph nodes, carotid arteries
Sitting position	Jugular veins, thyroid gland, trachea movements
	Lymph nodes—occipital, postauricular, preauricular, base of the skull) retropharyngeal, submandibular, submental
Carotid artery and Jugular veins	
Thyroid	Ask to swallow
Trachea	
Thorax, lungs	Ventilatory and respiratory function
	Key landmarks:
	Nipple
	Angle of Louis—2nd rib space
	Suprasternal notch
	Costal angle
	Clavicles
	Vertebra
Thorax	Anterior, lateral, posterior
Interior margin of scapula	7th rib
Orthopnea, dyspnea	
Crackles, rhonchi, wheezes, pleural rub	

Table 8.2: Patient's assessment chart

Patient's name:	Wd. No:
Address:	Reg. No. OPD:
Age:	I. P. D:
Sex:	Date of Admission:
	Date of Discharge:

Position	Standing/sitting/supine/dorsal recumbent/knee, chest, etc.
Draping	Draw sheet/top sheet/leggings/blanket
Body type	Strong/thin/obese/norms
Posture	Normal/limping/lordosis/kyphosis/deformity
Gait	Normal/limping/unsteady/stumping/tremors
Body movements	Normal/restricted/immobility
Hygiene and grooming	Clean/neat/unclean/infections
Dress	Well-dressed/hospital clothes/tight clothing
Affect and Mood	Calm/violent/aggressive/angry/sad/happy
Speech	Normal/slurred/inappropriate words/incompressive sounds
Client Abuse	
Substance abuse	Poison/excessive dose/drug/alcohol/any other
Vital signs	**Temperature:** Normal/low pyrexia/high pyrexia/hyperpyrexia subnormal/extremely cold
	Pulse: Normal/tachycardia/bradycardia
	Radial: Dicrotic/missing beat/feeble/not felt
	Brachial
	Temporal
	Respiration: Normal/dyspnea/orthopnea/difficulty in expiration/wheezing/rhonchi
	Blood Pressure: Normal/hypotension/hypertension
	Weight: Feet, inches, centimeter. Normal/less than/more than normal
Integument	**Skin:** Lesion/edema/melanoma/thickening/scaling/erythema/jaundice/induration/warts/wheels/flaking/moist/dry/hot/cold/sweating/pressure ulcers/crusting/abrasions/wound/infection/stretched/petechiae/purpura/pricks scar

Contd...

Contd...

Hair	Clean/dandruff/lice/nits/injury/alopecia/black/gray/brown/red/(white) dry/oily/short/long
Scalp	Integrity
Nails	**Color:** Pink/pale/blue/yellow/red/transparent/smooth/convex/concave, surrounding tissues smooth/without inflammation/inflamed/linear streaks or splinter hemorrhage/clubbing/Beau's lines/paronychia, koilonychia or spoon-shaped
Head	Circumference/size—normal/large/small
Eyes	**Eyebrows:** Normal/absent/movement possible
	Eyelids: Normal/ptosis/ectropion/entropion/redness/blink reflex
	Conjunctiva: *Bulbar*—white/red/yellow *Palpebral*—pink/pale/yellow
	Pupils: Equal/small/dilated
Ears	**External:** Pinna—Thick/thin/induration, external auditory—tenderness/discharge cerumen excess
	Middle ear: Hearing
Nose	**Shape:** Normal/deviated
	Size: Normal/enlarged
	Color: Pink/blue/black/red
	Deformity: Excoriation/polyps/sinusitis
Mouth	**Lips:** Pink/pale/blue/lesions/cracked/moist/dry/abraded
	Mucosa: Leukoplakia/cyst/ulcers/normal/whitish/gray/pink
	Gums and teeth: Pink/red/inflamed/bleeding/pus/lesions/dentures
	Tongue: Dull red/moist/slightly rough on top/smooth on lateral margins white/blue tip/dark red/moving all sides/tongue tie/glossitis
Palate	**Hard:** Normal/cleft/ulceration **Soft:** Normal/cyst/growth defect
Pharynx	Normal/infection/inflammation of tonsils
Neck	**Muscles**
	Lymph nodes: Enlarged/not soft
	Carotid artery: Normal/extended jugular veins
	Thyroid gland: Normal/enlarged trachea
	Movements: Normal/abnormal

Contd...

Contd...

Thorax	**Movements:** Lump/mass/tenderness
Heart	Palpitations/chest pain/discomfort/cough/fatigue/dyspnea/ edema feet/cyanosis/heart sounds
Breast	Normal/lump palpable/movable/discharge from nipple/flat nipple/cracked nipple/normal nipple
Abdomen	Peristalsis/absent
	Regions: Epigastric/hypochondriac Left/right—Lump; lumbar/umbilical/hypogastric/iliac
Extremities	Movements of joints
Upper shoulder	Flexion/extension/adduction/abduction
Elbow	Flexion/extension/rotation
Phalanges	Flexion/extension
Lower	**Hip:** Flexion/extension/adduction/abduction/rotation
	Knee: Flexion, extension, aduction/abduction/rotation
	Ankle: Medial rotation/lateral rotation/dorsiflexion

Abdomen (Table 8.3)

Table 8.3: Examination of Abdomen

1.	Inspection	**Linea Nigra:** Hypogastric region striae—lumber iliac region **Spider Nivae:** Umbilical region, operation scar All region shiny and thin skin contour—flat/round/oval Abdominal Girth—at the level of umbilicus—infection/injury/ ulcer
2.	Auscultation	Peristalsis—present/absent, Normal/abnormal
3.	Palpation	Lump/mass/soft/palpable liver/palpable—palpable/spleen not palpable
4.	Percussion	Fluid thrill/Hyman dull sound

Systemic Approach (Body System Approach)

Height: Weight
Time/temperature/pulse/respiration/blood pressure
Neurological: No known problem/oriented/disoriented/lethargic active/ comatose/muscular weakness/paralysis/headaches/seizures/vertigo/ syncope

Comments: Client is conscious, oriented. No headache.
Sensory deficit: Speech/tactile/pain/hearing/vision
Comments: All sensations are present. No deficit.
Musculoskeletal: No known problem
Comments: Muscle tone is good. No pain or weakness.
Integumentary: No known problem.
Skin: Intact. Color—Normal, Diaphoretic/dry, Temperature 99°F, drainage.
Comments:
Respiratory: Dyspnea, productive cough/nonproductive cough, character of respiration.
Normal/dyspnea/wheezing
Breath Sounds: Normal/wheezing/crepitations/rhonchi.
Comments:
Cardiac: No known problem. Angina—irregular rhythm, palpitations.
Circulatory—No known problem. Cyanotic/pain/varicosities/bleeding/edema/pulses
Comment:
Endocrine: No known problem. Diabetes, thyrotoxicosis, goiter.
Comments:
GI system: No known problem. Abdomen soft/tender/firm/distended. Nausea and vomiting present/diet/food allergies/diarrhea/normal bowel pattern/bowel sounds
Comments:
Genitourinary system: No known problem. Frequency/dysuria/hematuria/nocturia/dribbling/incontinence.
Comments:
Reproductive: Do you do monthly breast examination—yes/no
Testicular examination—yes/no
Changes noted:
Date of breast examination by physician:
Date of pap smear:
Breast: No change. Lumps/discharge/tenderness/abscess.
Comments:
LMP: Contraception
Gravida: Living/Para
No known problem: Tenderness/discharge
Itching Comments:

Functional Health Pattern Approach

- Health perception
- Nutritional/metabolic
- Elimination
- Activity and exercise
- Sleep and rest
- Cognitive/perceptual
- Self-perception
- Role, relationship
- Sexuality/reproductive
- Coping/stress tolerance
- Value/belief.

Human Response Pattern Appraoch

1. Exchanging
   - Cardiac
   - Cerebral
   - Peripheral
   - Skin integrity
   - Oxygenation
   - Physical regulation
   - Nutrition
   - Elimination
   - Safety.
2. Communicating
3. Relating
   - Relationship socialization
4. Valuing
   - Religious
   - Spiritual
   - Cultural.
5. Choosing
   - Coping
   - Participation
   - Judgment.
6. Moving
   - Activity
   - Rest
   - Recreation
   - Environment maintenance
   - Health maintenance
   - Self-care

- Meaningfulness
- Sensory perception.

7. Perceiving
   - Self-concept
   - Meaningfulness
   - Sensory perception.
8. Knowing
   - Current health problem
   - Health history
   - Current medications
   - Risk factors
   - Readiness
   - Orientation
   - Memory.

FORMAT FOR OBSERVATION, INTERVENTIONS

General appearance:
Critical/Acutely ill/Ambulatory/Disabled/Deformed/Conscious/Unconscious/Delirious/Violent/Aggressive/Collapsed
Vital signs:
Respiration: Regular/Irregular/Wheezing/Deep/Shallow/Cheyne-stoke/Apnea/Cyanosis/Choking/Dyspnea/Orthopnea/Crepitus/Rhonchi/Normal
Temperature: Centigrade/Fahrenheit
Normal/Subnormal/High pyrexia/Hyperpyrexia/Moderate pyrexia/Mild hypothermia/Deep hypothermia
Pulse—minute.
Regular/Irregular/Dicrotic/Bounding/Feeble/not felt/Tachycardia/Bradycardia/low volume
Blood Pressure—mm of Hg
Hypertension: Normal/Not recordable
Integuments: Skin: Intact/Injury/Wound/Scar/scabies/Ringworm/Allergy/Pigmentation/Hypopigmented patch/Induration/Urticaria/Ecchymosis/Purpura—cold and clammy/scaling—coarse/Toad-like/Orange pill/Hot/Pink/Red/Blue/Pale—vericose veins/yellow purpura
Wound: Incised/stabbed/crushed/contused/gunshot/superficial/deep/infected/clean/operated

Hair: Black/Red/White/Dye used/Clean/Dandruff/lice/Nitwits/Easily plucked
Scalp: Alopecia/Injury/Infection
Nails: Transparent/Pink/Smooth/Convex/Cuticles intact/Inflammed/Splinter/Hemorrhage/Beau's lines/Clubbing/Paronychia/Koilonychia.
Edema: Ankle/Prestibial/Abdomen/Back/Face/Anasarca/Pitting/Oozing.
Fracture: Skull/Ribs/Clavicle/Spine/Ulna/Radius/Femur/Humerus/Tibia/Fibula/Tarsal/Metatarsal/Phalanges/Carpal/Metacarpals/Phalanges/Pelvis.
Type of fracture: Simple/Compound/Complicated/Communited/Green stick/impacted
Sprints used: Bohler's/Thomas's/Simple/Cast
Bowel Movement: Normal/Painful/Regular/Irregular/Constipation/Diarrhea/Hemorrhoids/Fistula/bleeding/Melena/Peristalsis excessive/Normal
Micturition: Normal/Burning/Painful/Incontinence/Reflex in continence/Retention/Dribbling/Condom drainage/Indwelling catheter.
Bleeding: Wound/Operation/Incision/Eye/ear/Nose/Hemoptysis/Hematemesis/Rectal/Vaginal/Internal
Level of Consciousness:
Eyes opens spontaneously—to speech/to pain
Verbal Response—Oriented/Inappropriate words/Incomprehensible sounds/Motor response/Obey commands
Localized pain—Flexion withdrawl/Abnormal flexion/Abnormal extension/Flaccid
Reflexes: Blink reflex/Corneal reflex/Gag reflex
Airway: Clear/Secretions present/Tracheostomy/Endotracheal tube
Voice: Normal/Hoarseness/high/pitched
Speech: Slurred/Stuttering/Dysphasia/Normal
Heart: Sounds Normal/Extrasystole/Murmur
Abdomen: Soft/Hard/Tender/Painful
Verbal response: Oriented/can count/inappropriate words/incomprehensible sounds.
Motor response: Obeys commands/localizes pain/flexion withdrawal/abnormal flexion/abnormal extention/flaccid.

REVIEW OF LABORATORY DATA (TABLE 8.4)

Review Investigation Report

Table 8.4: Laboratory investigation report

1.	Hb percentage	:
2.	Urine analysis	:
	Specific gravity	:
	Albumin	:
	Sugar	:
	Bile pigments	:
	Acetone	:
3.	Urine culture	:
	Organisms present	:
	Sensitivity	:
4.	Blood cell count	:
	TLC	:
	DLC	:
	Platelets	:
5.	Blood sugar	:
6.	Blood urea creatinine	:
7.	Serum enzymes	:
	SGOT	:
	SGPT	:
8.	Serum electrolytes	:
	Na	:
	K	:
	Blood gas analysis pO_2, pCO_2	:
9.	Serum albumin	:
10.	X-ray and other reports	:
11.	CSF examination	:
12.	Other investigation reports	:
	ECG ECHO cardiogram	:
	LET, EEG, EMG Sonography, Biopsy, Audiometry	:

CHAPTER

9

Machinery, Equipment and Linen

AIM

Students know use of equipment and linen.

OBJECTIVES

- Students use linen, equipment properly
- Students maintain inventory
- Students know working and maintenance of machinery.

MACHINERY

Intravenous infusion pump (Fig. 9.1), ECG machine (Fig. 9.2), X-ray machine portable, nebulizer, defibrillator, ventilator (Fig. 9.3), cardiac monitor.

EQUIPMENT

Sphygmomanometer (Fig. 9.4), stethoscope, spirometer, cystoscope, laryngoscope, ophthalmoscope, sigmoidoscope, anesthetic trolley, dressing trolley and pulse oximeter (Figs 9.5 and 9.6).

DISPOSABLES

Intravenous infusion sets, syringes (Fig. 9.7), needles, gloves (Fig. 9.8), masks, caps, gowns, catheters, intracaths, urobag (Fig. 9.9), tracheostomy

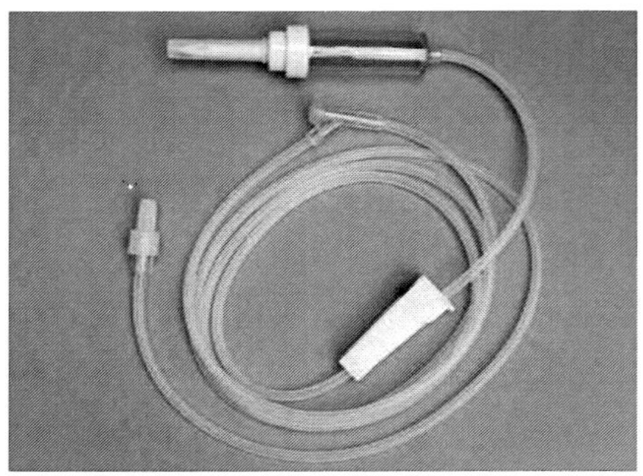

Fig. 9.1: Intravenous set

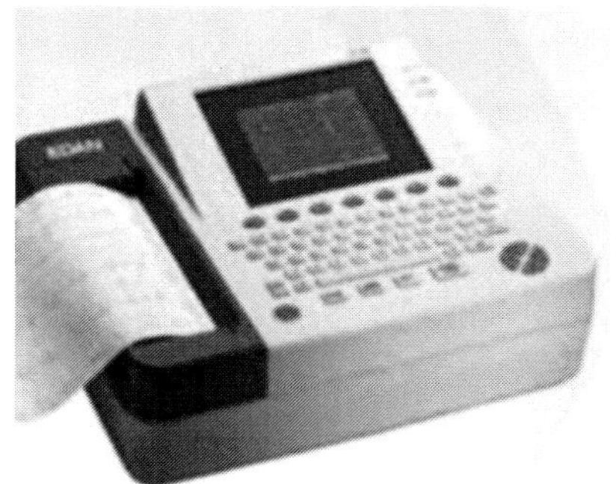

Fig. 9.2: ECG machine

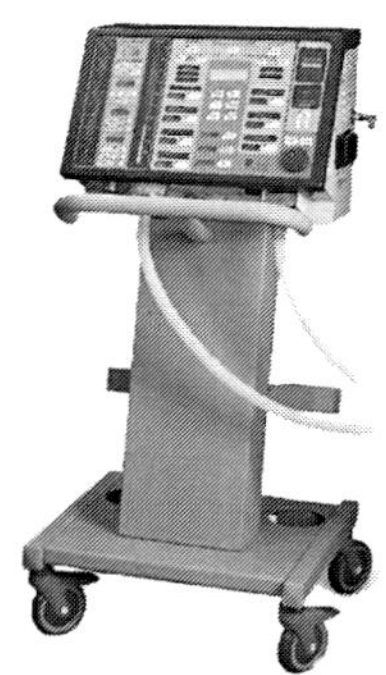

Fig. 9.3: Ventilator

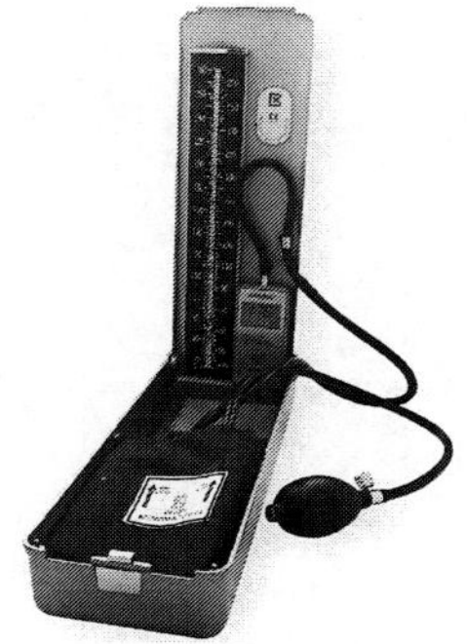

Fig. 9.4: Sphygmomanometer

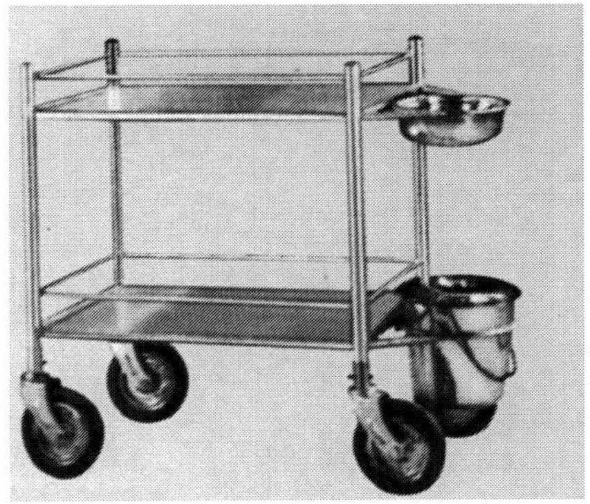

Fig. 9.5: Dressing trolley

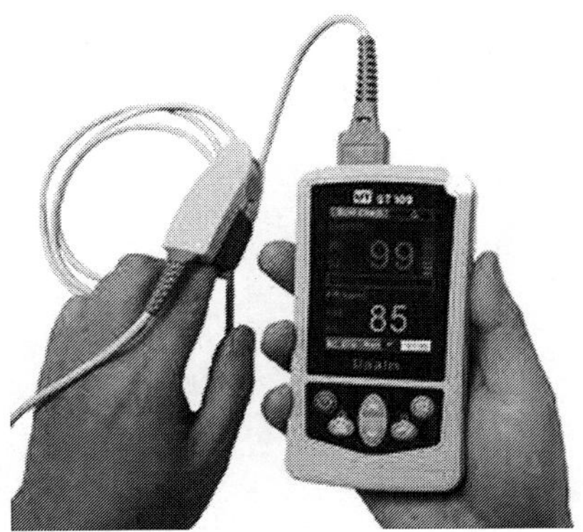

Fig. 9.6: Pulse oximeter

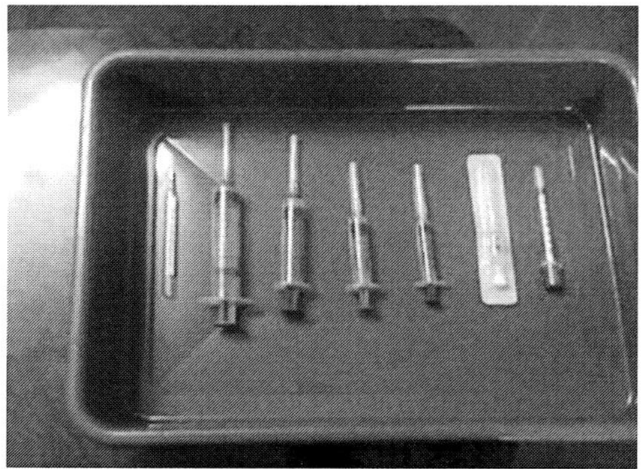

Fig. 9.7: Syringes

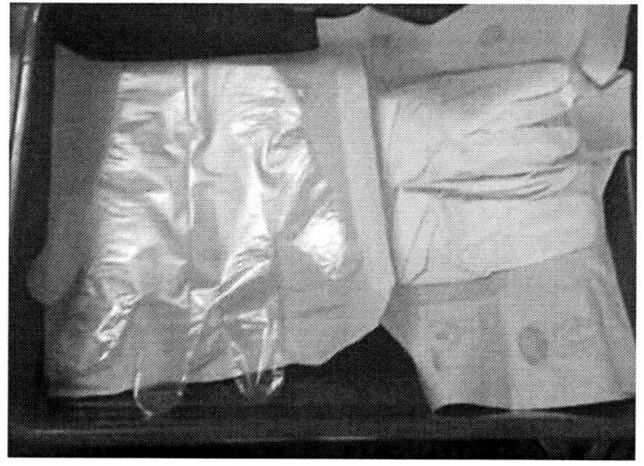

Fig. 9.8: Gloves

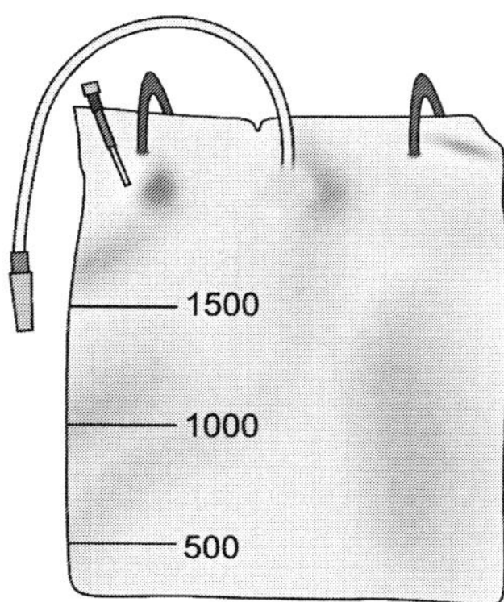

Fig. 9.9: Urobag

tubes (Fig. 9.10), colostomy bags, endotracheal tubes, drainage tubes and bags, plaster bandages.

FURNITURE

Bed, locker, overhead table, nurses station table, cupboard, trolleys, backrest stool or chair (Figs 9.11 and 9.12).

LINEN

Bedsheets, counterpanes, draw sheets, pillow covers, curtains, patient's clothes, gown, masks, leggings, drapes, hole towels, wash cloths/sponge bags, dusters, towels (face and bath), bath blankets, other blankets, hot water bag covers, ice cap covers, air cushion covers, elastic bandages, simple bandages, triangular bandages.

RUBBER GOODS

Mackintosh, catheters—plain, indwelling or self-retaining—Foley's, Malecot.

Ryle's tube (Fig. 9.13), drainage tubes, corrugated tube, hot water bags, ice caps, air cushion, tourniquet, air mattress, water mattress.

GLASSWARE

Ounce glass, drachm glass, thermometers—clinical and rectal (Figs 9.14 and 9.15), undine, test tubes, bath thermometer, lotion thermometer, urinometer, crockery.

PLASTIC

Trays, emesis basin, bedpans, urinals, enema cans, douche cans, inhalers, aprons, airways, tracheostomy tubes, basins, bowls, buckets, jugs, mugs, combs, toothbrush, droppers, catheters and tubes feeding cups (Figs 9.16 to 9.20).

METAL

Trays, dressing drums (Fig. 9.21), kidney trays (Fig. 9.22), needles, scalpel, instruments, dilators, retractors, speculum, tongue depressor, probe, forceps,

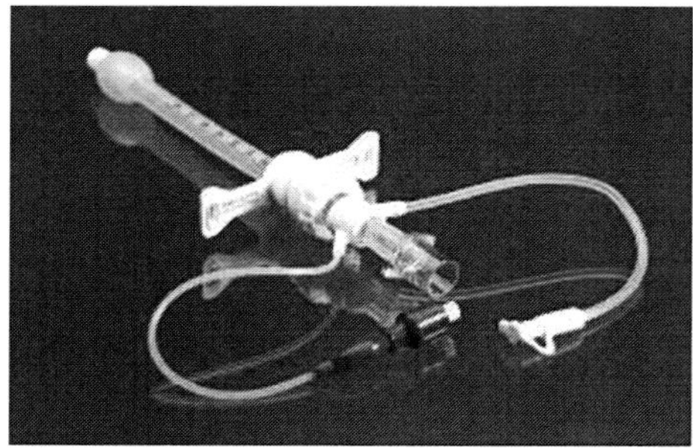

Fig. 9.10: Tracheostomy tube

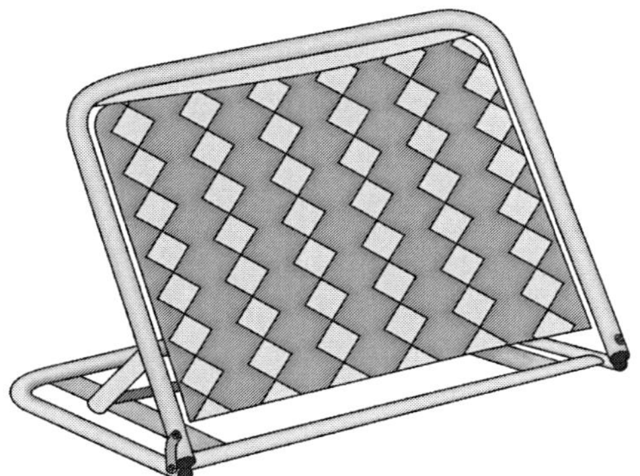

Fig. 9.11: Backrest

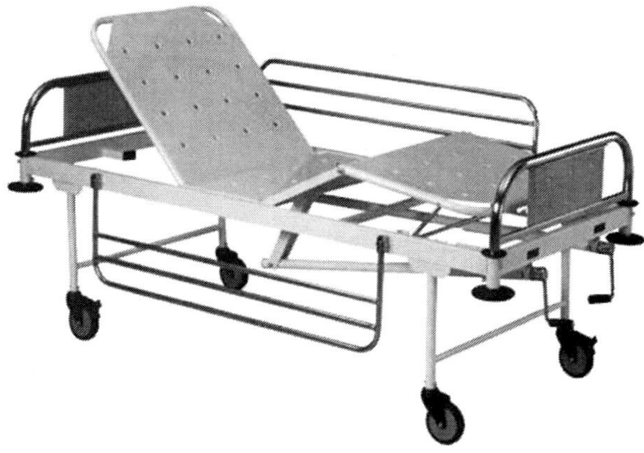

Fig. 9.12: Fowler's bed

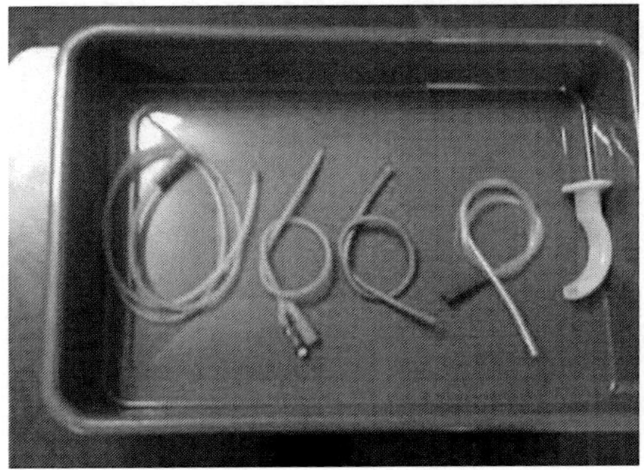

Fig. 9.13: Ryle's tube, catheters, airway

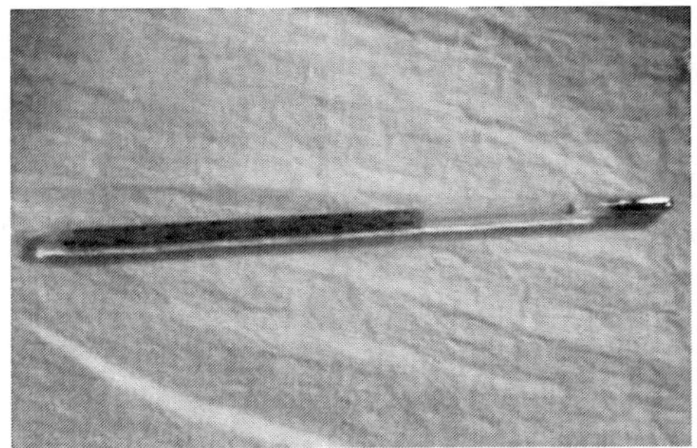

Fig. 9.14: Clinical thermometer

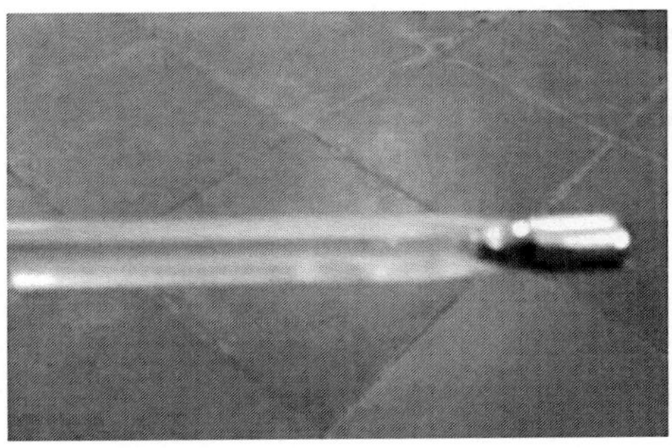

Fig. 9.15: Rectal thermometer

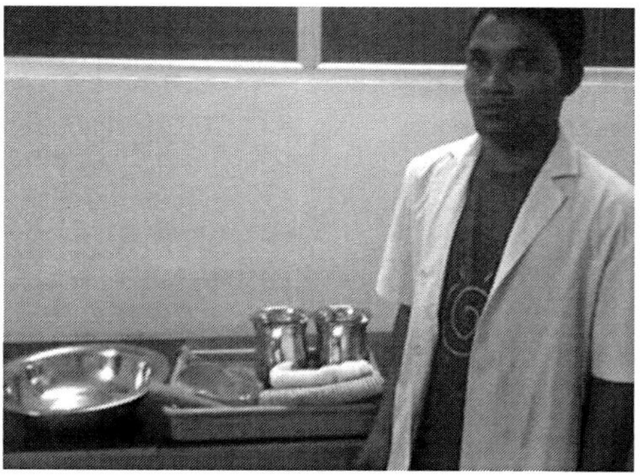

Fig. 9.16: Sponge tray

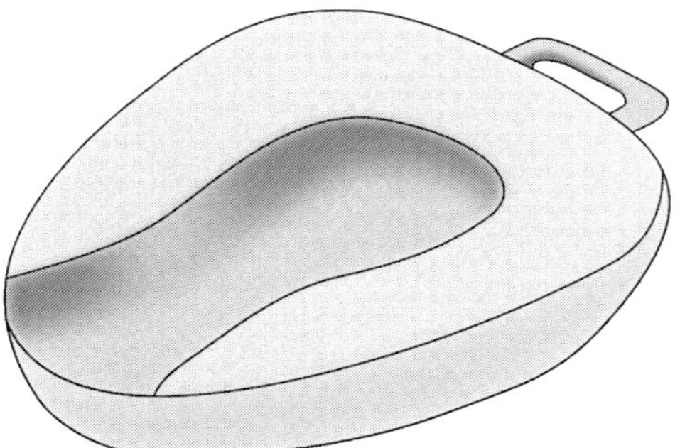

Fig. 9.17: Bedpan

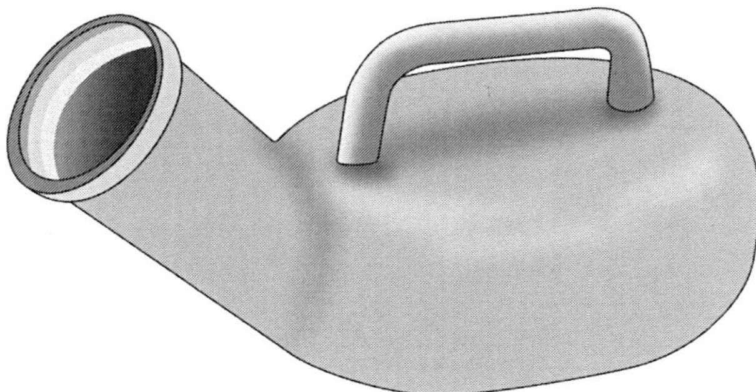

Fig. 9.18: Urinal

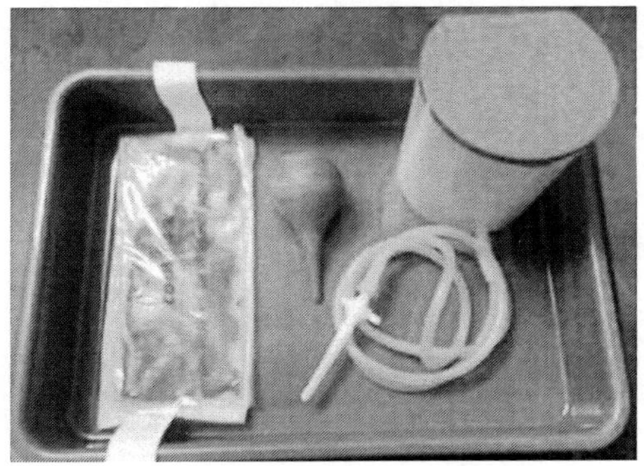

Fig. 9.19: Cool cap, douche can

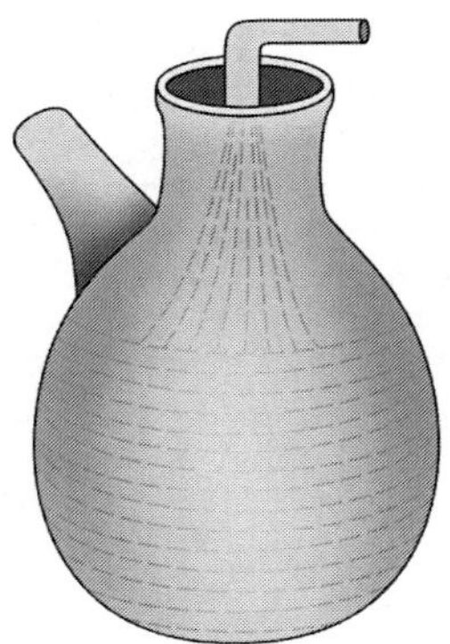

Fig. 9.20: Nelson's inhaler

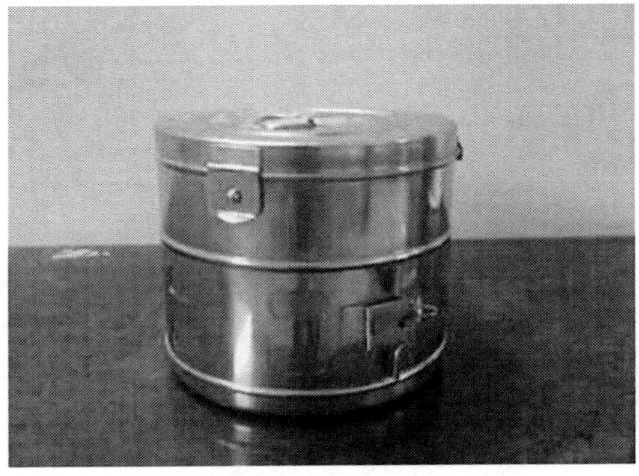

Fig. 9.21: Dressing drum

thumb forcep or dissecting forceps with and without tooth, hammer, towel clips, operation instruments, bowls, gallipots, suturing needles, cheatle forceps or utility forceps.

INDENT

Maintenance and Care (Table 9.1)

Table 9.1: Maintenance and patient's care

Name	*Use*	*Care*
Mackintosh	Used on bed to protect linen and mattress. Under the head in operation bed, routinely under the buttocks, while doing procedures like mouthwash (Fig. 9.23), dressing, enema under particular body part	It is washed with soap and water, dried in shadow or under the fan, wiped dry and powdered on both the sides and rolled and never folded when storing in cupboard after use
Catheters	Used to give oxygen, enema, remove urine from urinary bladder, oropharyngeal suction	Washed under running water, cleaned with soap and water and rinsed. Kept in long container after drying and powdering. When rinsing put water through one end and water should flow from other end if not, push air to remove block Disposable catheters are thrown into red disinfected container or red plastic bag (cat.no.7 in biomedical waste)
Ice cap, ice collar Hot water bag	Ice cubes are filled in ice cap and is kept on head to reduce body temperature, to prevent hemorrhage. It can be kept on other parts of the body like abdomen to stop internal hemorrhage, swelling. Ice collar is used around neck on to thyroid to reduce bleeding after operation. Hot water bag is used to keep the bed warm in admission and operation bed, to provide heat to the body part, to reduce pain, to increase body temperature in hypothermia	Washed with soap and water, wiped dry with soft cloth after keeping upside down for 10–15 minutes, powdered and air filled and closed with cap as air keeps two surfaces apart and prevents sticking together. To be kept away from heat source, sharps, as it may melt, if pierced

Contd...

Contd...

Name	*Use*	*Care*
Air cushion or air ring, air mattress, water mattress	Used under the buttocks to prevent pressure sore after air is filled. Air and water mattresses are used for patients to prevent pressure sore in unconscious, bedridden, very thin or obese patients	Wash with soap and water, wipe dry, fill air. Mattresses filled with air and water are wiped and dried on bed itself
Ryle's tube	Used for tube feeding, gastric aspiration (Fig. 9.24) Foley's catheter, Malecot's catheter—used as indwelling or self-retaining catheter in urinary bladder, 10 mL fluid is injected after inserting catheter through side opening to retain and when removing from bladder, fluid is aspirated first and then the catheter is removed	Washed with soap and water and rinsed, see for leakage, dry and powder. If infected, disinfect before washing
Glass articles—test tubes (Fig. 9.25), culture tubes	Used for testing urine for albumin, sugar, collecting swabs, sensation testing with hot and cold water	Washed with soap and water, Kept upside down on test-tube stand. Fill with cotton to prevent breakae, if not in use
Thermometers	Used for monitoring body temperature	Kept in plastic container after drying
Urinometer	Used to measure specific gravity of urine	Kept in a glass container provided along with or kept in box of thermocol
Sphygmomanometer	Used to monitor blood pressure of person	Lid is closed and kept after deflating cuff. Cleaned with savlon swab
Undine	Used for eye irrigation	Washed with soap and water, dried and wrapped in cotton or cloth and kept in box
Glass syringes	Previously used for injections, aspiration, irrigations, collecting blood samples	If used, wash with soap and water after separating barrel from piston. Wrap in gauze and send for autoclaving in dressing drum

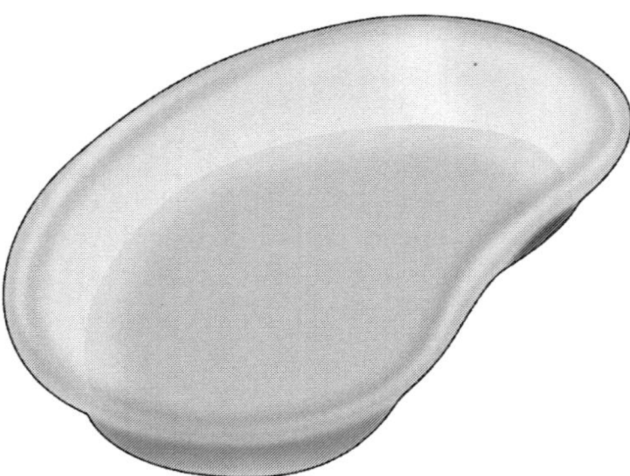

Fig. 9.22: Kidney tray

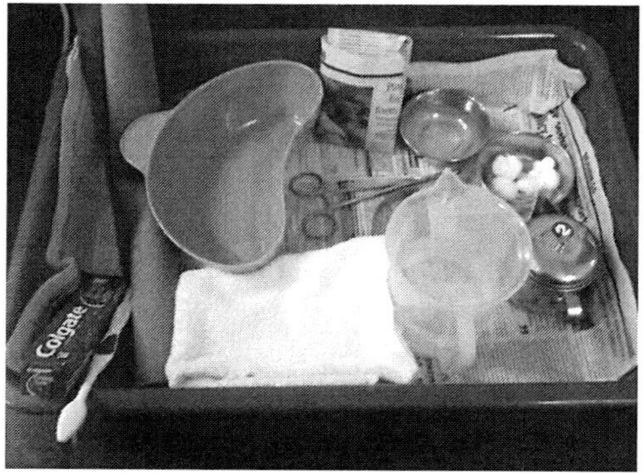

Fig. 9.23: Mouthwash tray

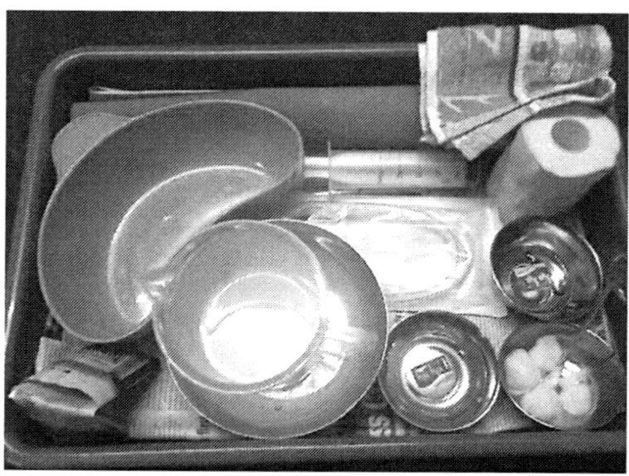

Fig. 9.24: Gastric aspiration tray

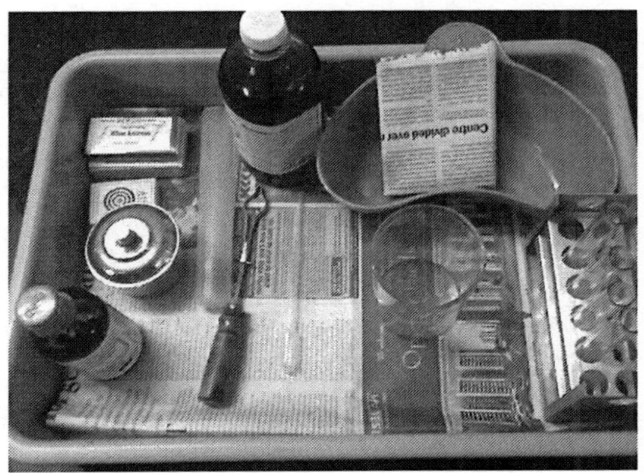

Fig. 9.25: Urine testing tray

CHAPTER

10

Meeting Needs of Patient

AIM

Students know the basic needs of client and assist in meeting those needs.

OBJECTIVES

- Students understand Maslow's hierarchy of needs
- Students plan care to meet client's needs.

MEETING NEEDS OF PATIENT

Basic needs: Activities of daily living (ADL).

The ADL requires physical ability, cognitive ability and safety. Physical ability is strength, flexibility and balance, accommodation for vision, hearing, touch, ability to recognize, judge and remember. ADLs are activities usually performed in the course of normal day. They are ambulating, eating, dressing, bathing, brushing teeth, grooming. Need for the assistance in ADL can be due to acute or chronic disease.

Patients with acute diseases, after operation require assistance for ADL and as they gain strength, progress through are less dependent on nurses for ADL activities. Chronic disease persists longer and may result in complete or partial disability. Hemiplegia, paraplegia, will need long-term assistance.

Need for assistance with ADL may be temporary, permanent or rehabilitative. Temporary assistance is for limited period. Irreversible spinal injury will require permanent assistance.

Fatigue, limitations in mobility, confusion, pain, are factors which make patient dependent on nurse for assistance in ADL. Assistance can change from day to day. Instrumental activities of daily living include shopping, writing, making phone calls, etc. which can be assisted by relatives, family, and friends.

MASLOW'S HIERARCHY OF NEEDS (FIG. 10.1)

Needs are generally more unconscious than conscious. Every person needs exist in different degrees and exist simultaneously. New needs emerge gradually. Lower level needs need not met completely before higher level needs can emerge. Maslow suggests that the degree of need satisfaction is positively related to mental health and that, theoretically, total need gratification and ideal health are synonymous.

Physiological Needs

First level needs are hunger, thirst, sleep and rest. Once physiological needs are satisfied, higher level needs emerge and when they are met new and still higher needs are recognized.

Safety Needs

Second level needs are safety needs. Protecting from extreme temperature, assault, murder, safety in natural disasters, wars, illness. When safety needs are satisfied need for love and belonging emerge.

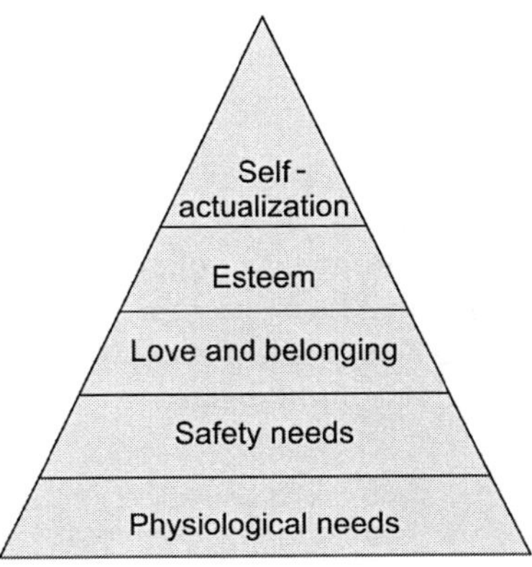

Fig. 10.1: Maslow's pyramid of needs

Love and Belonging Needs

Love is associated with sexual behavior and also with desire for affectionate relationship with people in general. Deprivation of this need results in loneliness and if severe, in major psychological disorder.

Esteem Needs

Desire for strength, achievement, adequacy, mastery, competence and independence. Unmet needs lead to inferiority, weakness and helplessness.

Self-actualization Needs

It is the highest level of need. It refers to persons continuously moving towards their highest potentials. Very few persons achieve this.

PROVIDING SAFE AND CLEAN ENVIRONMENT

Physical Environment

Room temperature is to be maintained from 20° to 22°C or 65° to 75°F. Air conditioning is the best method to control room temperature. Use of fans, coolers in hot climates and room heaters in cold weather help to maintain room temperature.

Light

Proper arrangement of artificial lights to natural light is not sufficient. It should not disturb patients. Night lights in bathrooms, darkness, rooms of children and old people helps to maintain safety by reducing risk of fall. Staircases and passages should be well-lighted at night.

Noise

Prevent noise from walking, moving trolleys, stretchers, and furniture. Loud noise, traffic noise should not enter the ward. Preventing dropping of articles and preventing noise while placing equipment. Silence is to be maintained in wards, and operation theater.

Humidity

About 40–60% humidity is comfortable. Humidifiers may be used when air is dry.

Ventilation

Ventilation means movement of air. It supplies fresh air and maintains humidity. Air in motion increases heat loss from body by radiation and improves circulation. Velocity of air should be from 15 to 45 ft/mn. Windows and doors should be kept open, use of fans and air conditioners help to maintain ventilation.

Esthetic Factors

Design, arrangement of room, color of walls, furniture contributes to esthetic factor, flower vase, pictures, curtains add pleasant look to room. Color of patient clothes, bed clothes, also helps to develop esthetic appearance. Unpleasant sites, bed pans, urinals, soiled linen, dressings should be removed immediately. To remove bad odors, room freshner should be used.

MAINTENANCE AND CLEANING PATIENTS UNIT

There may be separate rooms for patient with minimum furniture or the ward for many patients. Space needed for each patient is 50 square feet. If ward is of 30 patients, the area for patients should be 1500 square feet and additional space for toilets, store, utility room, pantry, washing room, dressing room of 1500 square feet.

Minimum equipment needed for each patient are bed, side table, locker, stool/chair, carpet, mattress, pillows, bedsheets, draw sheet, urinal, kidney tray or emesis basin, jug, glass, cup, drinking water, comb, paste, toothbrush, soap, soapdish, chart holders, waste papers, tissue papers. Control of pests, rodents, flies, bed bugs, etc. Dusting, sweeping, keeping toilets, sinks clean, and disinfecting floors and walls keeps pests, rodents, flies away. Bed making, changing linen, washing regularly, use of naphthalene balls, formalin tablets in cupboards prevent rodents and pests. Disposal of waste food, blood and body fluids properly prevents attracting rodents. Weekly washing, removing cobwebs, oiling equipment and hinges regularly, dusting helps to maintain cleanliness, prevents rusting. Equipment not required may be returned. Sending for repairing prevents storage of unnecessary extra-articles. Checking of cupboards, shelves, storerooms, cleaning and disinfecting, disinfecting beds, mattresses or keeping in sun, autoclaving and renewal prevents bed bugs. Keeping wards free of dust, dirt, excreted material, dressings, and blood keeps flies away. Dustbins should be foot-operated and kept closed.

REDUCTION OF PHYSICAL HAZARDS: FIRE, ACCIDENTS

Fall, accidents, poisoning, drowning, fire and burns are some of the physical hazards. Physical hazards contributing to fall can be minimized by adequate lighting in wards, and staircase. Obstacles in the environment can be reduced to minimum. Falls, burns, poisoning frequently occurs in bathrooms. Secure, easily seen grab bars and nonslip strips in front of toilet on floor will help to prevent falls. Medicines should be clearly marked when stored in cupboard. Outdated medicines should be discarded. Fire extinguishers should be installed. Protective grills over windows. Clients with visual, hearing, tactile and communication impairment should be given special attention and assistance. Side rails, trapeze bars, locking of wheelchairs, preventing slippery floors and bathrooms will create safety for clients.

Restraints

Restraints are used when other measures have failed to prevent immobilization for therapy as traction/IV infusion, nasogastric feeding, to prevent confused or combative client from self-injury, falling out of bed or wheelchair, to prevent a client from removing Foley's catheter, surgical drain or life support equipment and to reduce risk of injury to others by client.

Devices Used

- Jacket restraints—Vest or Posey
- Belt restraints
- Extremity restraints
- Mitten restraints
- Elbow restraints
- Mummy restraints.

Steps

Obtain doctor's order. Assess whether client needs a restraints. Review policy regarding restraints. Review manufacturer's instruction. Inspect area where restraint is to be applied. Assess condition of underlying skin. Explain to client and family the need of restraint. Attempt to obtain consent. Place client in proper body alignment. Pad skin and bony prominences before applying restraints. Apply appropriate restraints. Make sure that it is not over IV line or daily dialysis. Secure restrains with quick release tie. Insert two fingers under restrain. Observe every 30 mm for proper placement, skin integrity, pulse, temperature, color and sensation of restrained body part. Remove restrains for 30 minutes, every 2 hours. If client is violent remove one at a time. Apply proper size selected restraint, always refer to manufacturer's directions.

Jacket (Vest or Posey) Restraint

Apply jacket or vest over gown, *pajamas*, or clothes. Place clients's hands through armholes. Jacket restraints have sleeves. They close in back with zippers or hook and loop.

Vest restraints should have front and back of garment labeled as such. Secure vest according to manufacturer's directions. Some vests secure in the front of the client, and others secure in the back. Adjust to client's level of comfort.

Belt Restraint (Fig. 10.2)

Have client in a sitting position. Apply over clothes, gown, or *pajamas*. Remove wrinkles or creases from front and back of restraint while placing it around client's waist. Bring ties through slots in belt. Help client lie down, if in bed. Avoid placing belt too tightly across client's chest or abdomen.

Restrain client while lying or reclining in bed and while sitting in chair or wheelchair. Criss-crossing in back can cause risk of death from strangulation. Clothing or gown prevents friction against skin.

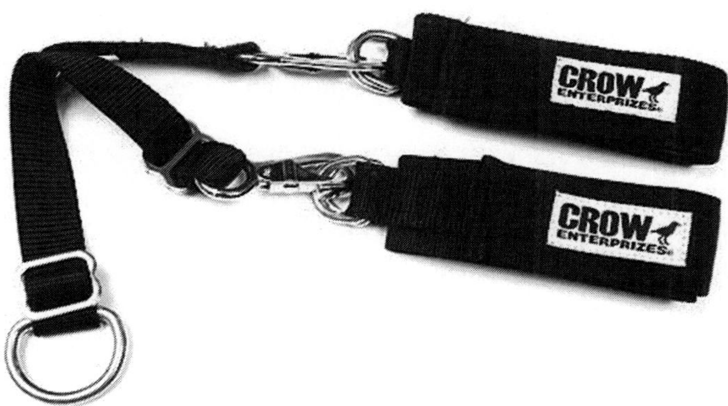

Fig. 10.2: Belt restraints

Restrains maintain center of gravity and prevent client from rolling off stretcher or sitting up while on stretcher or from falling out of bed. Tight application may interfere with ventilation. Lock the wheels, if present, for bed and wheelchair. Provide call bell within reach. Inspect for any injury.

Observe drainage tubes, catheters for correct positioning, provide appropriate stimulation and reorient.

Safe environment is one that minimizes falls, client inherent accidents, procedure inherent accidents, and equipment-related accidents.

Meeting basic needs of oxygen, nutrition, temperature and humidity can contribute to safe environment. Adequate lighting, hand hygiene, proper disposal of contaminated items creates safe environment. Use of restraints and side rails to prevent fall, preventing fire, poisoning, electrical hazards create safe environment. Supporting in bed and toilet for heavy and debilitated patients, safety in toilet, locks on beds and wheelchairs, call lights are safety measures in health setting. Check on crutches, walkers and integrity is required. Maintain outdoor walkways and stairs in good condition and free of holes, cracks and splinters.

Place disoriented clients in room near nurses station. Lock beds and wheelchairs when transferring. Electric equipment must be in working order and grounded. Seizures precautionary measures to be kept ready and protect patient from injury. Medical and surgical asepsis, food sanitation, insect and rodent control and appropriate disposal of human waste.

Typical hospital room has overbed table, bedside stand, chairs, lamp and bed. Hospital bed has firm mattress on metal frame that can be raised or lowered horizontally. Position of the bed can be changed by electrical controls incorporated into client's call light and in a panel on the side or foot of the bed. It saves energy and patient can change the position as he/she feels comfortable.

Adequate supply of linen to care appropriately is provided.

HYGIENE

Factors Influencing Hygienic Practice

Hygiene is the science of health and its preservation. Personal hygiene is individual measures taken to preserve one's own cleanliness and well-being.

Skin (Fig. 10.3)

Skin is an active organ and performs various functions, such as protective, secretive, excretory, temperature regulating and sensory.

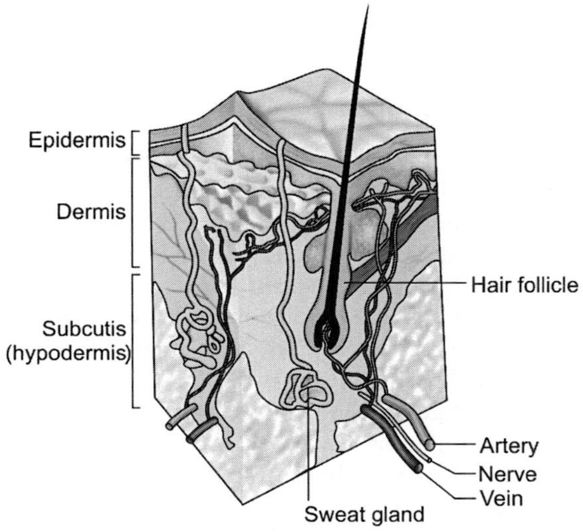

Fig. 10.3: Skin structure

Epidermis generates new cells to replace dead cells which are shed from outer surface of the skin. Dead skin may be source of bacteria. Normal bacterial flora prevents growth of pathogenic organisms. Sebaceous glands secrete sebum, an oily substance into hair follicle. Intact skin prevents entry of bacteria. Sweat glands secrete sweat to maintain temperature. Evaporation of sweat reduces body temperature. Salts and fluid is excreted through sweat. Perspiration and oil can harbor microorganisms. Bathing removes excess body secretions, reduces odor. Cleaning of skin removes dead skin and dirt.

Maintaining integrity, smoothness, hydration of oral mucous membrane is achieved by oral hygiene. Halitosis (bad breath) is also prevented by oral hygiene.

Intact skin protects body against injury and infection. When skin is cleaned, soaps and hot water are avoided. Soaps, alcohol-based lotions, alkaline residue causes drying. After cleaning, skin is completely dried and moisturizer should be applied to keep epidermis lubricated. Corn starch is dry lubricant which helps to reduce friction. Unicare, pericare are some water repellent ointments. Control or correct incontinence. Perspiration or wound drainage needs skin care. Absorptive pads and garments to be used for incontinence. Change of position relieves constant pressure on same area. Patient should sit on foam, gel or air cushion to redistribute weight.

Sponge Bath—Bed Bath

Bathing is a part of total hygiene. The extent of client's bath and method used, depends on the client's physical abilities, health problem and degree of hygiene required (Fig. 10.4, Table 10.1 and 10.2).

Assess the condition of the skin. Use lubricating soaps for dry skin. Assess the client's preference for frequency, time, type of hygiene products. Assess client's tolerance of activity, discomfort level, cognitive ability and musculoskeletal activities. Review orders for specific precautions regarding clients movement and positioning, e.g. tractions, surgery, fracture clients. Adjust room temperature and ventilation. Close room doors and windows, draw room divider curtain, screen the patient if in general ward and put of the fan near to bed. Prevent direct draft of air.

Prepare tray, offer bedpan or urinal, if needed. Provide towel and washcloth. Perform hand hygiene, if client's skin is soiled with drainage,

Table 10.1: Patient's physical ability and methods used for sponge bath

1.	Physically dependent	-	Special attention to skin assessment and provide care to prevent skin breakdown
	Or		
	Cognitively impaired	-	Total hygiene required, complete bed bath.
2.	Aged or dependent needing partial care	-	Partial bed bath
	Self-sufficient, bedridden clients who are unable to reach all body parts		Clean those parts which not cleaned

Table 10.2: Euipment used for sponge bath

Equipment tray	Wash cloths
Basins-2	Or sponge bags-3
Jug with hot water	Coconut oil or moisturizer
Jug with tap water	Starch powder
Soap in soap dish	or talcum powder
Bath blanket-1	Cologne water
Bath towels-2	
Face towel-1	

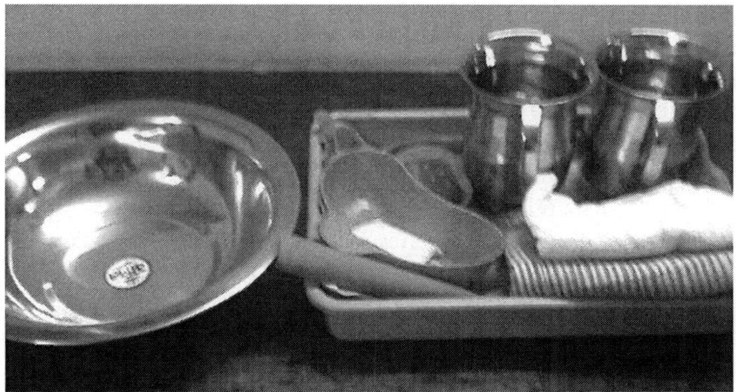

Fig. 10.4: Sponge tray

body secretions, apply disposable gloves. Ensure client is not allergic to latex. Bathe client complete or partial.

- Lower the side rail on right side of patient
- Assist to assume comfortable position
- Maintain body alignment
- Bring client closer to your side of bed
- Place bed at appropriate level
- Loosen top covers at foot of the bed
- Place bath blanket over top sheet
- Fold and remove top sheet underneath the bath blanket
- Use sheet when bath blanket not available
- If top sheet is to be reused fold and keep aside without touching to uniform. If not to be reused put in a laundry bag
- Remove clients gown or *pajama*. Start from unaffected side
- When IV drip is present, remove gown from arm without IV drip, lower IV container or remove from pump and slide the gown over the affected arm, over tubing and container. Rehang IV container, check rate or reset pump rate. Do not disconnect tubing
- Pull side rail up
- Fill wash basin 2/3 with warm water
- Ask client to place fingers in water to test temperature to tolerance
- Remove pillow and raise head 30–45°
- Place bath towel under client's head
- Place second bath towel over client's chest

- Immerse washcloth in water and wring it, if desired. Fold washcloth around fingers
- Wash client's eyes with plain warm water. Use different surfaces of wash, cloth to touch both eyes. Move from inner to outer canthus. Soak, if crust is present for 2–3 minutes before wiping
- Dry eyes thoroughly but gently
- Ask client, if soap is to be used on face
- Wash, rinse and dry well forehead, cheeks, nose, neck and ears
- Uncover arm near to you and place bath towel lengthwise under the arm
- Bath, arm with soap and water using long firm strokes from distal to proximal area (from finger to axilla), raise and support arm as required while wiping axilla
- Rinse and dry axilla thoroughly. If client uses deodorant, powder, apply it
- Fold bath towel half and lay it on bed beside client. Place basin on towel. Immerse clients hand in water to soak for 3–5 minutes before washing. Remove basin and dry hands
- Check water temperature and change, if needed
- Repeat same on the left side for left arm
- Cover chest with bath towel. Fold bath blanket to the umbilicus. Lifting towel edge away from chest, wash chest using long, firm strokes. Special cleaning under the breast in females. Keep chest covered between wash and rinse period. Dry well
- Put towel on chest, fold blanket to pubic region. Clean abdomen giving special attention to umbilicus, abdominal folds, stroke from side-to-side. Wash, rinse and dry
- Cover chest and abdomen with bath blanket. Expose one leg, keep flexed at the knees. Spread towel under the leg lengthwise. Place basin on towel and dip foot in basin to soak, if not possible simply wash with wash cloth. Use long firm strokes from ankle to knee to thighs. Dry well
- Raise side rail, move to left side, use same method for other leg
- Raise side rail, change water
- Lower side rail. Assist client in assuming prone or side lying position
- Place towel lengthwise along client's side
- Cover with bath blanket
- Wash, rinse, dry back from neck to buttocks using long, firm, strokes. Pay special attention to buttocks, sacrum, anus, give back rub, change water
- Apply disposable gloves if not applied
- Cover chest and upper extremities with towel and waist with bath blanket
- Expose middle portion only

- If client can wash cover entire body with bath blanket
- Provide perineal care
- Apply water repellent to area of moisture
- Dispose off gloves in receptacle
- Apply body lotion, if desired
- Assist client in combing hair
- Make client's bed
- Remove soiled linen in dirty linen bag
- Clean and replace bathing equipment
- Replace call light and personal possessions. Leave room as clean and comfortable as possible
- Perform hand hygiene.

Pressure Points, Pressure Ulcers and their Prevention

Back rub—3 minutes back rub. It promotes comfort, promotes relaxation, stimulates circulation and relieves muscular tension. Usually it is given after bed bath.

Contraindicated in burns, cardiac surgery, redness of skin, open wound, and vertebral fractures.

Equipment

Moisturizing lotion, BP apparatus, towel and blanket.

Explain the procedure. Adjust bed and comfortable position. Give prone position. Draw curtain, assess pulse, respiration, and blood pressure. Expose back, shoulders, arms and buttocks, cover other parts with bath blanket. Put towel alongside of back. Wash hands. Warm lotion in hands. Explain that lotion will feel cool and wet. Apply first to sacral area using circular movements. Stroke upward from buttocks to shoulders. Massage scapula with smooth firm stroke to upper arms and laterally along sides of back, down to iliac crest.

Do not lift hands. Continue for 3 minutes. Knead skin by gentle grasping and massage with long stroking movements. Wipe back with bath towel. Give comfortable position after clothing patient. Dispose soiled towel and wash hands. Reassess pulse and blood pressure.

Care of Nails

Feet and hand nails require special attention. Nail care involves soaking to soften cuticles, and layers of horny cells, thorough cleansing, drying and proper nail trimming.

Client with diabetes or peripheral vascular disease, no soaking is done as it causes risk for infection.

Equipment

Washbasin, emesis basin, washcloth, bath or face towel, nail clippers, orange stick, emery board or nail file, paper towels and disposable gloves.

Inspect surfaces of fingers, toes, feet and nails. Pay attention to areas of dryness, inflammation or cracking. Inspect between toes, heels, soles of feet.

Assess color and capillary refill of nails, note pulse. Ask females, if they use nail polish and polish remover frequently. See patient's age, case of diabetes, heart failure, renal disease, CVA, stroke to identify risks. Assess ability to care for nails, fatigue, and weakness. Obtain order, if policy of the hospital. Wash hands and arrange articles on overbed table. Pull curtain around bed, if necessary. If ambulatory ask client to sit in bedside chair, bedridden patient to supine position with head of the bed elevated. Place towel on mattress or mat on floor under patients' feet. Fill washbasin with warm water, test temperature, place basin and ask client to place feet in basin. For hands keep emesis basin on bed on towel. Ask client to dip fingers. Soak for 10–20 minutes. Rewarm after 10 minutes. Clean gently under the nails with orange stick while fingers are immersed. Remove emesis basin, dry fingers thoroughly. Clip finger nails straight across. Shape with file. If circulatory problem, do not cut only file. Put on gloves and clean feet with washcloth. Clean gently under nails with orange stick. Remove feet from basin. Dry thoroughly. Clean and trim toe nails. Do not bite corners of the toe nails.

Apply lotion to feet and hands. Assist client back to bed into comfortable position.

Remove disposable gloves and place in receptacle. Clean and return equipment to proper place. Record procedure and observations. Report any break in skin, induration, inform to nurse, incharge or physician.

PRESSURE AREA (FIG. 10.5)

Heels, sacrum, buttocks, elbow, shoulder, head, knee, and hip.

IMPORTANCE OF PERSONAL HYGIENE

Personal hygiene is important from point of view of comfort, safety and well-being. Proper hygienic care requires knowledge of scientific principles, integuments, oral hygiene, eye, ear, nose, anatomy and physiology.

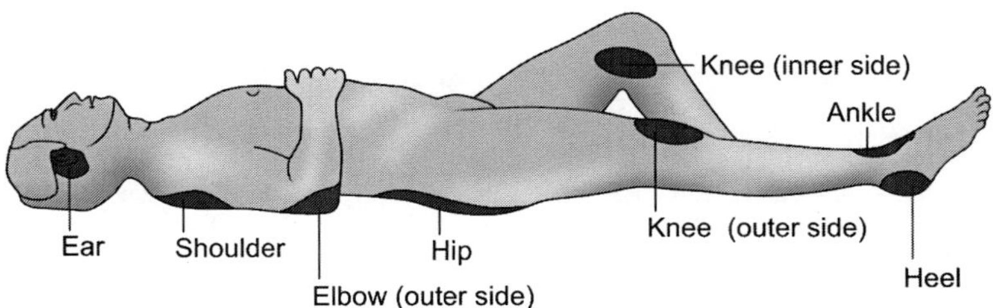

Fig. 10.5: Pressure areas

Cells require adequate nutrition, oxygen, fluids and hydration, good hygiene techniques promote normal structure and function of body tissues.

Personal hygiene maintenance prevents all infections due to microorganisms, fungus and infections.

CARE OF MOUTH: ORAL HYGIENE

Oral Cavity

Normally oral mucous membrane and tongue are moist normally pink. Injury, infection can be prevented through oral hygiene. Salivary secretion in mouth can be blocked by oral breathing, medications and exposure to radiation.

Purpose

- To maintain healthy state of mouth, teeth, gums and lips
- To remove food particles, plaques and bacteria from teeth by brushing and flossing
- To relieve discomfort resulting from unpleasant odors and tastes
- To enhance well-being and comfort
- To stimulate appetite
- To prevent parotitis—inflammation of salivary glands
- To prevent carries of teeth, stomatitis, glossitis, gingivitis and maintain integrity of lips, buccal mucosa, gums, palate and teeth.

Table 10.3 discusses about the oral hygiene for conscious and unconscious patients.

Equipment (Fig. 10.6)

Soft bristle toothbrush, nonabrasive fluoride toothpaste, dental floss, glass of water, emesis basin, face towel, paper towels, and disposable gloves.

Table 10.3: Oral hygiene for conscious and unconscious patients

Conscious patient	*Unconscious patient*
Wash hands and put on gloves. Inspect oral cavity, identify common oral problems remove gloves and wash hands. Prepare equipment at bedside. Raise bed to comfortable position explain the procedure. Place paper towels on overbed table and arrange other equipment at easy reach. Move client on side lying position. Place towel over chest. Apply gloves, apply toothpaste to brush, holding brush over kidney tray. Pour small amount of water. Hold brush at 45° angle to gumline. Brush inner and outer surface of teeth from gum to crown of each teeth	Wash hands. Put on gloves. Two nurses should provide care. One nurse actually cleans and other does suction to remove secretions. Open mouth with padded spatula kept at the back of teeth when patient is relaxed. Never use fingers to open mouth Perform mouth care every two hours. Protect from choking and aspiration. Give head turned to side position, lower the head end of bed and side rails. Explain the procedure, wash hands and put gloves. Place towel under patients head and emesis basin under chin position the patient.
Clean biting surfaces of teeth by holding top of bristle parallel with teeth and brushing gently back and forth. If patient assists, let him hold brush at 45° angle and lightly brush over surface and sides of tongue. Allow him to rinse mouth taking several sips of water. Allow him to gargle	Clean mouth using sponge toothettes moistened with hydrogen peroxide and water or swab moistened gauze. First, clean the inner chewing surface of the teeth and then the outer surface. Swab roof of mouth, gums and inside cheeks. Gently swab tongue, moisten swab with water to rinse. Repeat several times
Assist in wiping mouth. Allow him to floss. Allow to rinse mouth and spit in emesis basin or kidney tray. Assist him to comfortable position. Remove emesis basin, bedside table, raise side rail, lower bed to original position Wipe off overhead table, discard soiled linen and paper towels. Remove soiled gloves. Return articles. Wash hands. Wear gloves and inspect the condition of oral cavity	Do suction, if required. Apply thin layer of water soluble jelly to lips. Inform client that procedure is completed. Remove and dispose gloves. Place linen in proper receptacles. Wash hands. Wear gloves and inspect oral cavity. Assess respiration

HAIR CARE

Hair care matters with the person's appearance and feeling of well-being. Patient may not be able to take care of hair due to illness or disability. Immobilization may lead to tangling hair. Blood, antiseptics, sweat may soil the hair. Lice and nits may be troubling a patient. Proper hair care is required for patient's body image. Brushing, combing, shampooing are

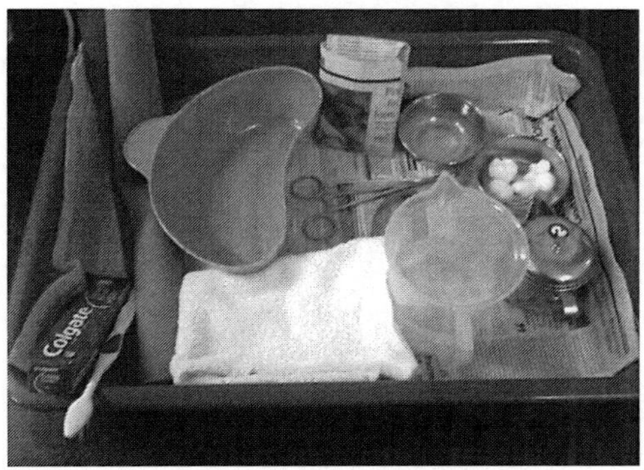

Fig. 10.6: Mouth care tray

basic hygiene measures for all the patients. Frequent brushing keeps hair clean and neat. Combing prevents tangling. When caring for patients with mobility problems, confusion, weakness preference for hair care practice, cultural preference may be taken into consideration. Long hair can become matted when patient is confined to bed. Scalp incision, laceration, blood, topical medication can cause tangling.

Hair should be combed and neatly groomed. Braiding can help to avoid repeated tangles. It should not be too tight so as to avoid bald patches.

Care of Hair

Position the patient comfortably. Place towel or piece of cloth under the hair, unbraid the hair. Apply hair oil. Separate each into two or more sections before application of oil. Comb gently removing tangles. Remove hair from comb with swab and place in paper bag, kept in kidney tray. Combing and brushing massages scalp and increases the circulation. Braid hair. Remove towel or piece of cloth, wash hands. Make patient comfortable and throw paper bag in dustbin.

Pediculosis Treatment

Put on gloves and wear gown. Keep piece of cloth under the hair on back. Remove tangles. Divide hair in sections and fasten the clip. Comb out from scalp to end of hair. Dip comb in water or clean with paper towel between each passing. Comb each section. Disinfect comb. Remove gloves after removing piece of cloth. Make patient comfortable.

Application of medicare shampoo and washing of hair can be done for lice treatment, if patient's conditions permits or no allergy present.

Shampooing of Hair

Equipment

Towels-2, Comb-1, Kidney tray-1, shampoo, bath blanket, mackintosh and draw sheet, or towel, hot and cold water in jug, basin and mug.

Positioning

Bring the shoulder on the side of the bed and place (trough is made by rolling the towel spread on mackintosh) through under the head keeping pillow, under the shoulder lowering the head. Keep bucket or washbasin at the end of the trough.

Pour hot and cold water to obtain warm water. Brush and comb patient's hair. Let patient hold towel or cloth over eyes. Pour water slowly with mug to wet hair. Apply shampoo. Work-up lather with both hands. Start at hairline and work towards back of neck. Massage scalp with finger tips.

Rinse hair with water. Make sure water drains into bucket or basin. Repeat rinsing till hair is free of soap. Apply conditioner or cream. Rinse again, wrap head in bath towel. Dry off moisture on neck. Dry hair and scalp. Use second towel, if needed. Comb hair and apply oil. Keep the patient's hair on towel placed on pillow, giving comfortable position. Place hot water bag to dry or use hair dryer.

CARE OF EYES, EARS, AND NOSE

Care of Eyes

Cleaning of eyes gently with wet swabs or washcloth from inner canthus to outer canthus. For unconscious patients, cleaning and instilling lubricating eyedrops will prevent dryness of cornea.

Cleaning of eye glasses should be done carefully and protect from breakage. Lens should be cleaned with special solutions. Artificial eye may be cleaned with warm normal saline.

Care of Ears (Fig. 10.7)

Clean ear with moistened end of washcloth, rotated gently into ear canal. When cerumen is visible, retract ear lobe and wax may come out. Never use sharp objects to remove wax.

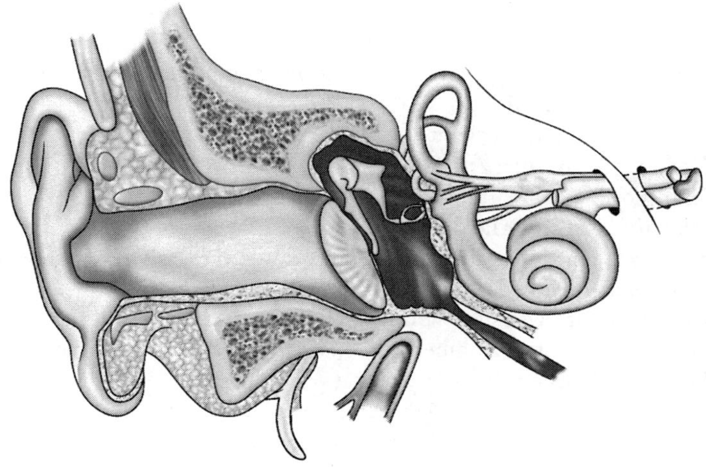

Fig. 10.7: Structure of ear

Irrigation is required, if impacted cerumen is present and it is done with order from physician. Instill three drops of glycerin at bed time to soften wax and three drop of hydrogen peroxide twice a day.

Warm water syringing removes loosened wax. Place mackintosh and kidney tray under the ear, positioning the patient sitting or side lying with affected ear up. Gentle irrigation directed at the top of canal removes wax. Wipe off moisture and observe ear canal.

Care of Nose

Gentle blowing into tissue paper by patient will remove secretions. Using wet washcloth or cotton will remove nasal secretion. Gentle suctioning can be done, if excessive nasal secretions are present.

Eyes: Administration of Eyedrops

Equipment

Medication bottle with sterile eye dropper or ointment, cotton swabs, warm water and washcloth and clean gloves.

- Check order
- Identify client
- Assess condition of eye
- Determine any known allergy

- Determine any visual alteration
- Assess knowledge regarding medication
- Assess knowledge regarding medication therapy and desire to self-administer medication
- Explain procedure to client
- Wash hands, arrange articles
- Wear gloves
- Ask patient to sit or lie down
- Hold swab on client's cheek bone, press downward, ask him to look up
- Hold medicine filled dropper 1–2 cm hyperextended
- Soak crust with wet swab. Clean eyelids above conjunctival sac
- Drop the prescribed number of drops into the conjunctival sac
- If patient blinks or closes eye, repeat procedure
- Ask patient to close eyes lightly. For ointment, apply thin stream of ointment evenly along inner edge of lower lid from inner to outer side. Ask patient to close eye and rub lightly with cotton swab, if not contraindicated.

PATIENT ENVIRONMENT: ROOM EQUIPMENT AND LINEN—MAKING PATIENT BED

Room Equipment

Typical hospital room contains minimum furniture like overbed table, bedside stand, chair, lamp, bed, telephone, water jug, glass is kept on bedside stand or locker. Call light, TV set, wall mounted blood pressure gauge, oxygen and vacuum wall outlets, personal care items. Special mattress and bed boards. Comfort and positioning equipment. Bed provides safety, adaptability. Firm mattress on metal frame that can be raised or lowered. Bed contains safety features such as locks on the wheels or casters. Side rails prevent fall.

Bed/cot/metal rod/spring/wood/plastic wire

Length: 78"—195 cm—6 ½ ft.

Breadth: 38"—95 cm—3.2 ft.

Height: 28"—70 cm—2.4 ft.

Mattress/cotton/coir/foam/dunlop/air/water

Length: 76"—190 cm—6.4 ft.

Breadth: 36"—90 cm—3 ft.

Bedspread/top sheet

Length: 3 meters—108"

Breadth: 2 meters—72"
Mackintosh—waterproof rubber or plastic
Length: 3 ½ ft. from shoulder to knee to be placed 9" below from heel end to knee level.
Draw sheet—drawn from side-to-side
Length: 150 cm 60"
Breadth: 110 cm 40"
Pillow
60 cm × 45 cm × 10 cm
Cotton foam
Pillow cover 62 cm × 48 cm
Space between two cots: 3–3.5 ft, 36"–42", 90 cm–105 cm
Sizes of cot mattress and linen.

Bed Making

Principles

- Avoid pulling of bed linen. Lift mattress to loosen bed clothes
- Fold linen from head end to foot end
- Arrange linen in correct sequence with closed end of folded sheet away from you
- Do not put soiled linen on floor. Place in dirty linen box or laundry bag
- Do not let the uniform touch bed linen or bed
- Use clean and dry bed linen
- Dust mattress and turn upside down
- Wash hands before and after bed making
- Keep open-end of pillow cover away from entrance
- After completing bed making see that locker, chair, stool are clean and in order and in line
- When making occupied bed try to avoid unnecessary movements of patient, cot and shaking
- Stand on one side, complete half bed then to other side. Save time and energy.

Types

- Simple open bed
- Occupied bed
- Admission bed
- Operation bed

- Fowler's bed
- Cardiac bed
- Rheumatoid bed
- Renal bed
- Amputation bed
- Divided bed.

Open Bed (Fig. 10.8)

- Collect articles and keep linen in sequence on chair at foot end.
  Articles required: Kidney tray, duster, mattress 1, pillow 1, wet mop, bed sheets 2, blanket 1, counter pen 1, mackintosh 1, draw sheet 1, pillow cover 1.
- Wash hands. If bed is already made, loosen the top linen from head end and proceed to foot end. Remove only by one folding in six. Bring lower third over middle third and upper third over lower third. Fold at the center towards you. Place over chair. Fold draw sheet. Roll mackintosh. Place over chair. Turn mattress. Dust mattress with duster. Unfold bottom sheet lengthwise. Keep center of the sheet at the center lengthwise. Keep 10" at both ends extra and miter the corner at head end. Face head of the bed, place hand away from head of the bed under top corner of mattress and lift with other hand, tuck top edge of bottom sheet under mattress. List up top of edge of sheet 18" down from top and lay it on top of mattress to form triangle.

Tuck lower edge of sheet which hangs down under the mattress. Hold remaining part of sheet covering the edge of mattress. Tuck under mattress.

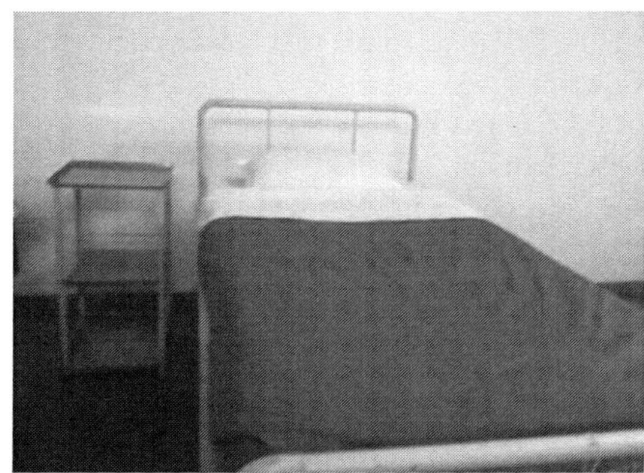

Fig. 10.8: Open bed

Move towards foot end keeping sheet smooth. Lay mackintosh and draw sheet and draw sheet rolled. Tuck one side under the mattress. Raise side rail, if present and go to other side. Do the same way as on the right side. Place top sheet, blanket, counterpen. Turn top sheet edge, on edge of the blanket. Tuck top linen at the foot end under mattress, keep pillow with cover at the head end.

In closed bed, top clothes are tucked at both ends and in open bed corners are folded from one side to allow the patient to get into bed.

Occupied Bed

When making occupied bed turn patient to one side. Place folded (lengthwise) sheet, mackintosh, draw sheet on right side—tuck at the top, right side and bottom. Turn patient to right and complete the tucking of sheet and draw sheet on left side. Cover the patient by placing top sheet, blanket and counterpen folding edge of top sheet on blanket and tucking at the foot end or folding and tucking at the bottom, if patient does not require the blanket.

Admission Bed (Fig. 10.9)

Make a simple open bed. Place top sheet and blanket. Fold 9" on both sides.

Tuck under the mattress on right side. Fold the corners from both sides to make a broad rectangular. Fold in the center of bed lengthwise to keep 2/3 part of the mattress covered.

When patient comes, remove tucked top linen and cover the patient. Unfolding it and tuck at the foot end. It is easy to receive the patient, if

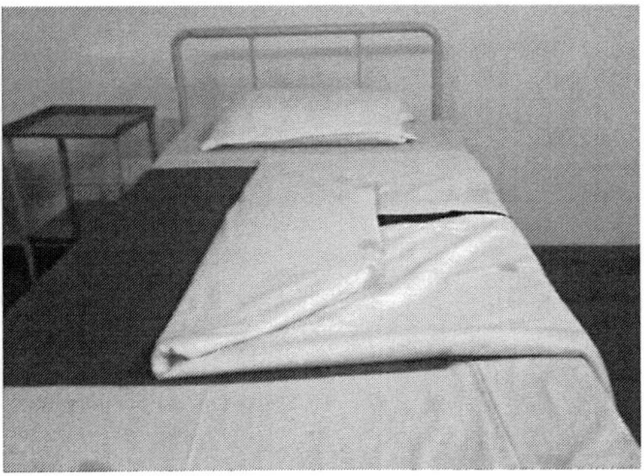

Fig. 10.9: Admission bed

top linen is side folded, and keeps the bed warm. Place two hot water bottles in winter season to keep bed warm.

Operation Bed

When client is sent to operation theater, operation bed is prepared to receive him in surgical ward after operation. Place bed spread or white sheet on mattress. Place mackintosh and draw sheet in the middle. Place small mackintosh and towel or draw sheet removing pillow. Fold top linen that is white sheet, blanket and couterpen 12" on head side and 12" on foot side. Tuck on one side and leave open one side (towards ward's entrance) folding in triangular manner. Fold till midline. Place hot water bag to keep bed warm in winter season. Keep ready saline stand, thermometer kidney tray, oral care tray, and suction.

Fowler's Bed (Fig. 10.10)

It is bed with few modifications like raising of head and back. Patient can sit with support or we can make use of backrest and pillows on plain simple bed. Bolster is placed under knees for comfort. Patient with dyspnea feels better with this bed. Postoperatively patient can sit with support.

Cardiac Bed

Make a simple bed. Raise head end 30° or support with a backrest and extra pillows. Place cardiac table in front of the patient. Modern beds have

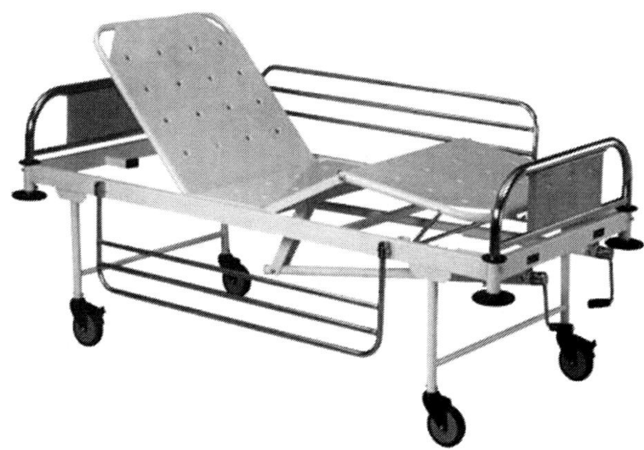

Fig. 10.10: Fowler's bed

the arrangement of side table which can be used for various purposes. Patient can rest his arms and head on a pillow. If not available, place a cardiac table and a pillow.

Rheumatoid Bed

Use of extra blanket and sand bags to support the swollen joints.

Renal Bed

To increase the perspiration, extra blanket underneath is used but as there are drugs, dialysis, its use is not of importance and practiced.

Amputation Bed

Put mackintosh under the part, support with two sand bags.

Divided Bed

Two parts of mattress are present in this bed. Double sets of sheets are used to cover two halves of mattress. Its use is not practiced.

COMFORT

Importance

Comfort is described as subjective state in which there is sense of physical and psychological well-being with freedom from pain, want or anxiety.

Comfort can be achieved through relieving pain, soft clothes, mattress, pillows, bolsters, cushions, appropriate positions, backrest, heart table, relief from pressures from within and outside, elimination, maintaining room temperature and body temperature, meeting needs of nutrition and oxygen and relieving distress.

Identifying Communications

Nonverbal Communications

- Restless, crying, moaning
- Unusual quietness, withdrawal
- Unusual position
- Facial expressions
- Change in color and temperature

- Increased or decreased respirations
- Nausea, vomiting
- Excessive perspiration
- Insomnia, behavioral changes.

Comfortable room temperature (18°C–21°C) well-ventilated, minimum noise, proper lighting is to be provided to patients. Drafts are to be avoided and patients positioned away from windows. For older adults extra blanket for warmth. Infant needs light blanket. Bed and mattress should provide support and comfortable firmness. Extra pillows are required for positioning. Soft cotton clothes should be worn. Keep bed clean and dry. Fowler's position, lateral positions may sometimes required for comfort supporting dependent parts to protect pressure points and helps in relaxation. Emptying of bladder will relieve discomfort and enhances rest.

Relief from Pain

Pain is protective physiological mechanism. Stimulus for pain can be physical or mental in nature, whereby damage may be actual tissues or to person's ego. Pain is tiring and demands energy, pain changes person's behavior. Pain is leading cause of disability. Pain is of three types, (i) acute, (ii) chronic, (iii) malignant or cancer pain.

Other types are nociceptive (somatic or visceral) and neuropathic. In nociceptive pain, there are four processes— (i) transduction, (ii) transmission, (iii) perception and (iv) modulation.

Transduction: Pain producing mechanism begins in the periphery when stimulus sends an impulse across the nerve fiber. Nerve fiber enters spinal cord via dorsal horn route and travels ending in gray matter of spinal cord. Once transfusion is complete, transmission begins.

Thalamus nerve cells—cerebral cortex in brain interprets the quality of pain through past experiences, knowledge, cultural association in perception of pain. Cell damage results in release of pain producing substances. Damage may be thermal, mechanical or chemical origin. Pain producing substances are bradykinin, potassium, serotonin, histamine. These substances surround nerve fiber, extracellular fluid, spread message and cause inflammatory response. These are called neurotransmitters. After the pain, impulse ascends the spinal cord and thalamus transmits information to higher centers in the brain. Brain interprets quality of pain.

Transmission: Nerve fibers of two types conduct painful stimuli. Myelinated A—delta fibers and unmyelinated—C fibers. 'A' fibers send sharp, localized and distinct sensations and detect intensity. 'C' fibers impulses are poorly localized, burning and persistent.

Common factors that disrupt normal pain reception include trauma, drugs, tumor growth, and metabolic disorder. Transmission can also be affected by neuroregulation. These substances are in dorsal (posterior) horn cells of spinal cord at nociceptor, at nerve terminals and in spinothalamic tract. Neuroregulators are of two types—(i) neurotransmitters, (ii) neuromodulators. Neurotransmitters send electric impulse across the synaptic cleft between two nerve fibers which are excitatory and inhibitory in nature. Neuromodulators increase or decrease the effect of neurotransmitters, e. g. endorphins.

Perception: It gives meaning to pain.

Soma to sensory cortex—location and intensity.

(Precentral gyrus)

Association cortex—feeling about pain.

Limbic system—sensation of pain.

Gate control theory: Cells in spinal cord, thalamus, limbic system regulate the pain impulses by regulating or blocking them. Pain impulses pass through when gate is open and blocked when gate is closed. Closing of gate is basis of pain relief. Massage stimulates mechanoreceptors which are thicker, and faster.

Modulation: Process of inhibiting or changing pain impulses. Neurons from brainstem to dorsal anterior horn cells of spinal cord release substance such as serotonin, norepinephrine, endorphins which inhibit the transmission of pain and help to produce analgesic effects. Factors influencing pain are age, gender, culture, meaning of pain, attention, anxiety, fatigue, coping style, family and social support, measures to relieve pain are change of position, pacing, rocking, rubbing, eating medication, application of heat or cold to painful site, muscular activities, verbal methods (prayer) cursing, concentration exercises, acupressure, acupuncture, chiropractic, etc. Analgesic are most common method of pain relief. Opioids, nonopioids, adjuvants such as sedatives, antianxiety agents and muscle relaxants enhance pain control and relieve other symptoms.

Patient controlled analgesia (PCA). These are portable infusion pumps containing chamber for syringe or bag that delivers small, preset dose of medication. Most pumps have locked safety systems to prevent tampering. Local and regional anesthesia, epidural analgesia is also used to relieve pain.

Positioning: Positions used for comfort, rest and sleep are:

- **Dorsal recumbent:** Lying in bed on back with knees slightly flexed and supported with pillow
- **Left lateral:** Patient lies on left side keeping left leg straight and right leg flexed at knee supported on pillow

- **Right lateral:** Patient lies on right side with right leg straight and left leg flexed at knee and supported with pillow
- **Fowler's position:** Bed head raised to 30° or patient supported with backrest and pillows, knees flexed and supported with bolster or pillows
- **Cardiac position:** Patient sits in fowler's position with cardiac table or overbed table in front and supported by soft pillow.

SLEEP

Sleep involves a sequence of physiological status maintained by highly integrated central nervous system activity that is associated with changes in peripheral nervous, endocrine, cardiovascular, respiratory and muscular system.

Phase I: Nonrapid eye movement (NREM) has four stages.

Stage I: Lasts for few minutes. Decreased physiological activity begins with gradual fall in vital signs and metabolism, person is easily aroused.

Stage II: Period of sound sleep. Relaxation progresses, stage is 10–20 minutes but still can be aroused. Body functions continue to slow.

Stage III: Initial stages of deep sleep, difficult to arouse. Muscles are completely relaxed, vital signs decrease, but are regular (15–20 minutes duration).

Stage IV: 15–30 minutes. Deepest stage of sleep.

Phase II: Rapid eye movement (REM)—90 minutes after sleep has begun. Rapidly moving eyes, fluctuating heart and respiratory rates, increased or fluctuating blood pressure, vivid full color dreaming may occur. Loss of skeletal muscle tone, very difficult to arouse. Duration of REM increases with each cycle average being 20 minutes. Each person passes through 4–6 complete sleep cycles per night. NREM 1-2-3-4 NREM 4-3-2- REM NREM 2-3-4- NREM –4-3-3-2-REM.

Sleep Requirement and Pattern

Neonates to 3 months of age—16 hours/day—40–50 minutes cycle wakening, eyes open, vigorous sucking, REM sleep 50%, hunger, pain, cold causes urging (Table 10.4).

Factors Affecting Sleep

Physiological, psychological and environmental factors affect sleep. Drugs and substances can affect sleep. Milk, cheese, meat, help to sleep. Medications prescribed can lead to more problem than benefit. Lifestyle,

Table 10.4: Sleep requirement and pattern for children

Toddlers preschoolers	–	12 hours/day, REM 20%
School age	–	9–10 hours/day, REM 20%
Adolescent adults	–	7 ½ hours/day, REM 20%
Old age	–	No stage 4
Neonates to 3 months of age	–	16 hours/day, 40–50 mn cycle, wakening, eyes open, vigorous sucking, REM sleep 50%, hunger, pain, cold causes urging
Infants	–	15 hours/day, REM, 30%

sleep pattern, emotional stress, environment can affect sleep. Noises in hospitals, hospital bed, sleeping alone, close proximity of patients, noise from ill, confused patients, lights in wards may disturb sleep. Exercise and fatigue, food and caloric intake also affect weight loss or gain can also affect sleep.

To Promote Normal Rest and Sleep

Assess the sleep pattern. See whether patient has any pre-existing health problem, change in lifestyle anxiety, excitement, anger, situational crisis, etc. Follow bedtime routine and bedtime environment, if possible. Reduce and control noise, light, other factors, provide warmth, cleanliness, extra blankets if needed, loose clothes, firm mattress dry and soft bedsheets, and glass of milk.

Hot applications may help to promote sleep. Extra pillows, change of position, face wash, back rub may also help.

Sleep Disorders

- Insomnia
- Abnormal sensation, movements in sleep
- Excessive day time sleepiness
  - Intrinsic sleep disorders—disorders of initiating and maintaining sleep
  - Extrinsic sleep disorders—developing from external factors
    - Psychiatric sleep disturbances
    - Neurological sleep disorders
    - Medical disorders.

Insomnia: It is a symptom. It consists of chronic difficulty in falling sleep, frequent awakening from sleep, short sleep, insufficient quantity and quality. It may be due to physical or psychological reason.

Temporary insomnia may be due to stress such as work, family problems. Between situations client is able to sleep well.

Insomnia is often due to poor sleep habits.

Sleep apnea: Lack of air through air passage for 10 seconds–2 minutes.

It may be obstructive, central, or mixed type. Treatment of cardiac and pulmonary diseases, emotional problems solutions will help.

Narcolepsy: It is central nervous system (CNS) dysfunction of regulation of sleep. Day time feeling sleepy.

Cataplexy: Sudden muscle weakness during anger, laughter. Client may fall by losing voluntary muscle control.

Parasomnia: These produces undesirable physical symptoms due to autonomous nervous system changes and skeletal muscle activity during sleep in older children. Somnambulism (Sleepwalking) night terrors, nightmares, enuresis, teeth grinding may be seen.

NUTRITION

Importance of Diet in Health and Illness

Body needs energy and anabolic substance which is received through consumption of food.

Tissue repair, organ function, normal balance, water electrolyte balance, kinetic energy requirement are met through intake of protein, carbohydrates, fats, minerals, vitamins and water.

Carbohydrates are the main source of energy, 1 g gives 4 calories, glucose is used for brain function and for muscle actions.

Proteins are needed for body tissue growth, maintenance and repair. Collagens, hormones, enzymes, immune cells, DNA and RNA are composed of proteins.

Essential amino acids are those amino acids which cannot be synthesized and only received from diet. Complete proteins are high quality protein from animal source.

Negative nitrogen balance occurs when body loses nitrogen, in burns, fevers, starvation, head injury, trauma and infections.

Linoleic acid is essential for human being.

Linolenic acid and arachidonic acid can be synthesized in body. Water content of body is 60–70% of body weight, fluid needs are met by ingestion of fluids, waters foods, fruits and vegetables and output is from perspiration, urine elimination.

Patient may require more fluid or restriction of fluids. Normally 5–6 liters. Vitamins are essential for normal metabolism.

Vitamin A, D, E and K are fat soluble and B complex and vitamin C are water soluble. Fresh fruits, vegetables, sunlight, fish oil, citrous fruits, yellow fruits and vegetable provide vitamins.

Minerals are micronutrients which are necessary Ca, K, Na, chlorides, Fe, Co, Cu, etc.

Factors Affecting Nutritional Needs

Metabolism refers to all biochemical reactions in cell. Increased metabolism in goiter requires more calories. Rest and minimum work will only need minimum calories. Starvation, metabolic disorders will result in wasting of body. Anabolism is building of complex substances and catabolism is breaking down to simpler substance. Newborn infant, preschooler require food for growth and development and their requirement of protein, vitamins, calcium is more as growth and development continues. Growing children need calories from 1500 to 3000/day. Pregnant woman will need extra diet for fetal growth.

Digestion: Patients with gastritis, have problem of digestion. Easily digested foods, liquids will be their requirement. Roughage is avoided in these conditions.

Absorption: Absorption may be affected in various conditions like malnutrition, postoperative period, GI tract diseases, malabsorption syndrome. Temporary modification of diet is necessary. Food is absorbed in the intestines by passive diffusion, active transport and pinocytosis.

Socioeconomic status: The type of food a family can afford and eat will depend on its socioeconomic status. Advice regarding low priced nutrition, food is necessary to plan family diet.

Psychological factors: Anorexia nervosa, bulimia nervosa of refusal and eating of large amount of food, both are abnormal food habits. Environment, cooking process, appetite affect food consumption.

Health status: Nutrition less than body requirement or over weight, obese person's nutritional needs will be different. First category will need high caloric, high protein diet whereas other will require less diet. Disease conditions requires special type of diets. Patient with diarrhea requires replacement of fluids and food which is easily digested, hypertension condition creates need for reduced salt intake. Diabetic patient has to control the intake of carbohydrates. Liver diseases, fat is prohibited and rice sugar diet is given. Deficiency may be reduced by diet therapy.

Assessment of Nutritional Status Variables

- Anthropometry
- Laboratory tests
- Diet and health history
- Clinical observation
- Client expectations.

Anthropometry: Measuring size and make-up of body.

- Height
- Weight—same time of the day, same scale, same clothing
- Rapid weight gain—fluid shifts, compare height and weight relationship for clients with renal failure and congestive cardiac failure, weight gain of 2 pounds is significant. It means there is retention of 1,000 mL fluid
- Ratio of height to weight
- Mid upper arm circumference
- Triceps skin fold comparison is made with the standard
- Body mass index = $\dfrac{\text{weight (kg)}}{\text{height in meters squared (Ht m)}^2}$
- >25—upper boundaries of healthy weight
- >35—at risk of coronary heart disease, diabetes, some cancers, hypertension
- BMI between 25 and 35—over weight
- >30—obesity

Laboratory test:

- Fluid balance
- Liver functions test
- Measuring plasma proteins—albumin, transferrin
- Hb and iron binding capacity.

Check albumin level in chronic diseases.

Check Prealbumin level in acute diseases.

Albumin levels are affected in hemorrhage, draining wounds, burns, steroid therapy, stress, surgery and dehydration.

Nitrogen intake = total proteins ingested in 24 hours.

Dietary History and Health History: Client's habitual intake of foods and liquids, preference, allergies, ability to obtain food, religious food patterns, socioeconomic status, consumption of alcohol, drug and general nutrition knowledge.

Clinical Observation (Table 10.5)

Table 10.5: Clinical observation related to dietary and health history

Risk for aspiration, gag reflex, swallowing
Edema, hydration of mucous membrane, signs of dehydration
Anemia—pallor tongue, lips, nails, conjunctiva
Bitot spots
Dermatitis, weakness nausea, anorexia, vomiting, diarrhea, aphasia, peristalsis, urine sugar and albumin, presence of jaundice, stomatitis, tender calf, breathing difficulty, oral hygiene, pharyngitis, fever, exophthalmos, goiter, disease condition

Client's expectations: Developing nutrition plan with client, use of teaching material and knowledge to meet client's expectations.

Serving and Feeding Helpless Patient

Equipment: Towel, plate, spoon, feeding cup, straw, glass of water, napkin and kidney tray.

- Check the orders for prescribed diet
- Create pleasant environment
- Position the patient. Draw overbed table
- Help him to wash hands and face, gargle
- Put towel over chest
- Wash hands
- Talk pleasantly
- Cut food to small pieces of mouth size and serve one piece at a time
- Encourage to take variety of foods
- Give enough time to chew and swallow, do not hurry
- When sufficient quantity is fed, stop feeding and give glass of water by feeding cup or straw
- Help the patient to wash his face and hands
- Dry face and hands
- Make patient comfortable
- Take all articles to utility room and discard waste. Clean articles or put then in receptacle for plates, spoon and fork. Clean feeding cup, kidney tray and clean with soap and water, dry and keep it back or boil it. If infected, paper plates, plastic spoons, disposable glass, paper napkins also can be used and then disposed off.

POLICIES AND PRACTICES IN RELATION TO SERVING DIET

Diet is planned for every patient as per his requirements, disease condition, food habits and on time.

Create a pleasant environment at the time of eating. Room should be well-ventilated, quiet, decorated and attractive surroundings and cheerful atmosphere.

Giving bedpans and urinals, painful treatments cleaning, treatments, dressings, doctor's round, disturbances to be avoided at food time and should be over one hour before the food is served.

Soft music helps to create cheerful atmosphere.

Walking patients can come to dining room for food. Sitting on stool or in bed with overbed tabel or Fowler's position, if required, will provide patient some comfort and change to increase appetite and food tray can be placed to feed conveniently.

Meals should be served in clean, covered container.

Provision for washing of hands and face before and after meals is to be made.

Oral Diet

When patient is sick, diet is prescribed according to his need and disease condition.

Soft, easily digested foods, nourishing fluids and therapeutic diet are prescribed. Therapeutic diets consist of:

- Full diet
- High protein diet
- Low caloric diet
- Low residue diet
- Low fat diet
- Salt restricted diet
- Rice sugar diet
- Butter milk diet.

In anemia, iron containing foods are advised.

Small and frequent feeds are prescribed in emaciated patients, post-operatively, children and gastric disorders.

Extra fluids about 5–6 liters per day are included in patients with fluids—deficit in cases of fever, diarrhea and urinary problems.

Fluid and sodium is restricted in patient with cardiac problems, hypertension, ascites. In liver diseases, fat is restricted. Porridge, egg preparations, custard and jelly, etc. are appetizing foods used for emaciated, underweight patients and with problems of GI tract. When oral food is contraindicated nutritional requirement is met with parenteral food.

Unconscious patients, patients with aspiration, regurgitation problem enteral catheter is passed and liquids are given through drip. Patient with peptic ulcers milk drip is given.

Nasogastric Feeding

Tube may be passed into stomach or jejunum.

Gastric feeding is done in patients with risk of aspiration. If there is risk for aspiration, feed is given through jejunal tube. Nasogastric or orogastric tube may be used for feeding (Table 10.6). Feeds are started with 20–50 mL/hr and increased 25 mL every 12 hours.

Procedure

Collect the articles in a tray and place conveniently near bed.

Explain the procedure to patient and ask him for cooperation and what he is suppose to do when inserting a tube. Put towel around neck.

- Wash hands
- Clean the patient's nostril (left) with swabstick dipped in normal saline or soda bicarbonate. Put in paper bag
- Wash hands and wear gloves
- Apply lubricant to tip of Ryle's tube and direct into the (left) nostril medially and to the backward direction (Fig. 10.11)

Table 10.6: Indications and requirements for nasogastric feeding

Requirements	*Indications*
Tray containing tube—check the tube for patency, holes, cracks, elasticity, measure the distance from nose to ear and mark on tube and for ear to zippy sternum 10"–12"	Cancer of GI tract, head and neck trauma, critical illness—intestinal inflammation—mild pancreatitis—inadequate oral intake, CVA brain, neoplasm, convulsions, unconsciousness, patients who refuse food.
Feeding cup with water syringe 20 mL. Ryle's tube—Levin's tube in a bowl. Water soluble jelly or liquid swab stick. Saline in small bowl. Kidney tray, paper bag, gauze pieces. Gloves, glass of water	

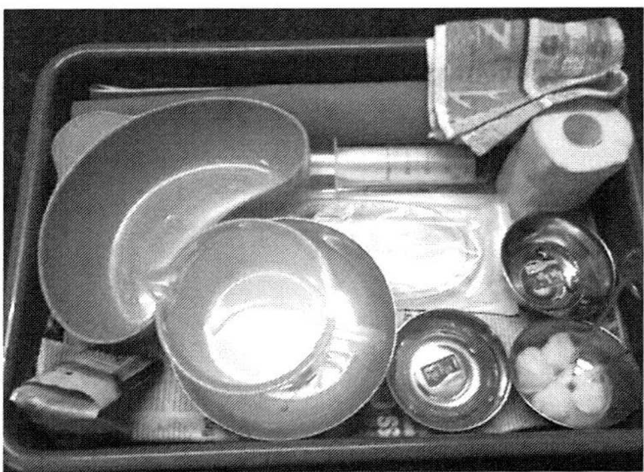

Fig. 10.11: Ryle's tube feeding tray

- Ask the patient to swallow the tube. See that it is not coiled up in mouth. Insert slowly and ask patient to swallow, advance the tube as he swallows
- Confirm that it is in stomach by aspirating. Fluid will come from tube
- Fix the tube on nostril and forehead, if used for feeding, aspiration for longer duration
- Aspirate and feed 10 mL of water through barrel of syringe to clear the tube, make sure tube is in the stomach or intestine and then feed 200–250 mL feed, strained and some water after the feed. Close the tube fasten the end to patient's forehead
- Make patient comfortable
- Chart feed type/time and amount on input/output chart
- Remove articles and clean and dry and keep back in proper place

When clients with gastroparesis, that results in esophageal reflux, at risk for aspiration pneumonia. Tube is placed beyond the stomach into intestine.

Small bore feeding tubes create less discomfort. Size is 8–12 Fr and 36–43 inches long. Stylet is used during insertion of small bore tube to stiffen it. Stylet is removed when the correct position of the feeding tube is confirmed.

Equipment

Disposable feeding bag and tubing or ready to hang system. 30 mL or larger leverlock or catheter tip syringe. Stethoscope, ph indicator slip, infusion pump.

Procedure

- Assess client's needs for enteral feeding, e.g. impaired swallowing, decreased level of consciousness (LOC), head or neck surgery, facial trauma, surgeries of GI tracts
- Auscultate for bowel sounds
- Verify physician's order for formula, rate, route and frequency
- Explain procedures to patients
- Wash hands
- Prepare feeding container to administer formula temperature 37°C. Connect tubing to container, fill container with formula or feed
- Give patient high Fowler's position
- Determine tube position by aspirating gastric content, measure pH and observe appearance
- Initiate feeding
- Pinch proximal enclosure of feeding tube, remove plunger from syringe and attach barrel to tube
- Fill syringe with measured formula, release tube and hold syringe high enough to allow empty it by gravity, refill, repeat till prescribed amount is delivered to patient. Give 150–200 mL, increasing 50 mL per feed
- If to be given by continuous drip, hang feeding bag and tubing on IV pole and connect distal end to the proximal end of feeding tube
- Connect tubing through infusion pump and set rate
- Advance tube feeding gradually in tube 300–400 mL
- Administer water after formula
- Cap or clamp the proximal end of feeding tube when tube feeding not administered
- Monitor input/output and chart
- Record amount, type of feed, patency of tube and client's response.

Gastrostomy Feeding

Equipment

Feeding container or ready to hang bag, 30 mL syringe, infusion pump, pH indicator strip, stethoscope and clean gloves.

- Assess the need for feeding
- Auscultate peristalsis
- Verify order for formula, rate, route, frequency
- Perform hand hygiene
- Assess gastrostomy site for breakdown, irritation, drainages

- Explain procedure to client
- Prepare feeding formula
- Have feed at room temperature
- Connect tubing to container
- Shake formula well. Fill tubing full with formula
- Elevate head 30–45°
- Wear gloves and verify tube placement
- Attach syringe and aspirate gastric secretion observe and check pH. Return content to stomach. If more than 100 mL, do not give feed and inform doctor
- Flush with 30 mL water
- Initiate feeding.

With Syringe

Pinch proximal end of gastrostomy tube, remove plunger, fill syringe, release tube and elevate. Refill it till whole formula is given.

Continuous Drip

Hang container to IV pole, clear air from tubing, connect tubing to gastrostomy tube, begin feeding at prescribed rate. Give water between feedings. Clamp proximal end, assess skin around tube exit site, wash hands, replace equipment, record feed given.

PARENTERAL NUTRITION

Parenteral nutrition is form of specialized nutrition support where nutrients are given intravenously. Aseptic precautions, careful assessment is required. It is given in cases of head injury, burns and sepsis.

Lipid Emulsion

It is given to provide calories and essential fatty acids. They can be given through peripheral or central line by Y connector tubing.

Three-in-one Admixture

- Ten percent dextrose, amino acids and lipids. They are usually given in large veins (subclavian) (superior vena cava)

- After catheter placement, catheter is flushed with saline or heparin and position is radiologically confirmed
- Central venous catheters (CVCs) are sutured in place with sterile dressing
- Before beginning infusion, verify order and inspect solution
- Infusion pump is to be used. 40–60 mL/hr is given. Rate is gradually increased and is usually given at night so that client can move at day time
- Complications can be infection, metabolic acidosis, pneumothorax
- Intravenous fluids like dextrose 5%, normal saline, ringer lactate administered to provide minimum caloric requirement, fluid and electrolytes.

URINARY ELIMINATION (FIG. 10.12)

Review of physiology of normal urinary elimination.

Normal Urinary Elimination

Kidneys (glomerulus) filtrate urine from blood. About 99% of it is reabsorbed and 1% is excreted as urine. In 24 hours, output of urine

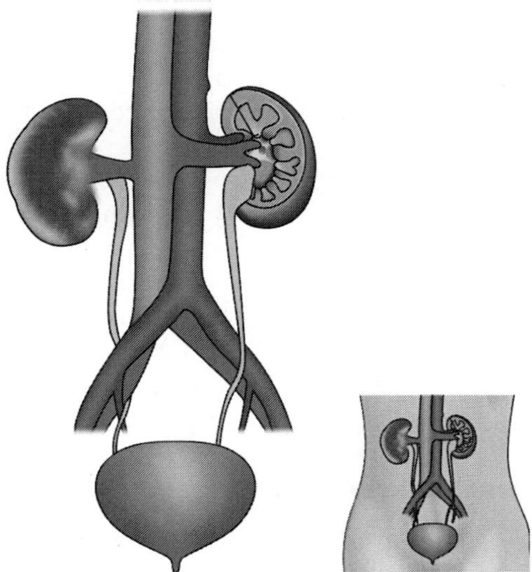

Fig. 10.12: Urinary system

is 1,500–1,600 mL. Output less than 30 mL per hour indicates renal failure.

Bladder can hold 600 mL of urine. Person may sense desire to urinate when content of bladder are 150–200 mL. Detrusor muscle of bladder contracts when person voids and the urethral sphincter relaxes.

Composition and Characteristics of Urine (Table 10.7)

Table 10.7: Composition of urine

Water 96%	Sodium—6 g
Solutes 4%	Chlorides—7 g
	Calcium—0. 2 g
Urea—20–30 g	Potassium—2 g
Uric acid—0. 6 g	Phosphates—1. 7 g
Creatinine—1. 2 g	Sulfates—1. 8 g

Characteristics

- **Quantity in 24 hours:** 1,000–1,500 mL
- **Color:** Amber or pale yellow
- **Odor:** Aromatic
- **Specific gravity:** 1,010–1,020, increased when solutes are increased and abnormal presence of sugar and albumin.
- **pH:** 6 reaction acidic. Blue litmus turns red. It is transparent, on standing cloudy.

Abnormal constituents: Sugar, blood, bile salts, bile pigments, crystals, acetone, ketone bodies, sediments cloudy and foamy.

Abnormal color	–	Red, dark color, smoky, yellow, orange.
Abnormal odor	–	Fishy, sweet, ammonia.
Reaction	–	Alkaline sometimes on eating leafy vegetables.
Oliguria	–	500 mL/24 hours.
Anuria	–	No urine is secreted.
Polyuria	–	Large amount more than 1,800 mL for 24 hours.

Factors Influencing Urination

Volume and composition of urine and patients ability to urinate is influenced by many factors:

- Pathophysiological conditions
- Slowing or hindrance in physical activities

- Lack of privacy
- Muscle tone of abdominal and pelvic floor
- Fluid balance
- Surgical and diagnostic procedures
- Cognitive, physical and functional factors resulting in retention, incontinence and infection
- Renal dysfunction.

Alterations in Urinary Eliminations

Prerenal Alterations

Decrease in blood flow to and through kidneys resulting in oliguria, anuria in cases of dehydration, starvation, congestive cardiac failure.

Renal Alterations

Causing injury to glomeruli and renal tubule, e.g. transfusion reactions, glomerulonephritis, diabetes mellitus.

Postrenal Alteration

Obstruction to the flow of urine due to calculi, blood clots, tumors, enlarged prostate, nerve lesions. Joint diseases and parkinsonism. It is difficult to reach toilet on time.

Uremic Syndrome

There is increase in nitrogenous waste, altered regulatory functions, and in severe uremic symptoms renal replacement therapies are needed.

Dialysis and organ transplant are two methods of renal replacement. Dialysis is of two types peritoneal and hemodialysis.

When damage occurs to spinal cord above sacral region there is loss of voluntary control of urination but reflex pathways are intact and urination occurs reflexively. The condition is called as reflex bladder. Prostatic enlargement hinders bladder emptying and retention occurs. Decrease in renal function produces oliguria. If urine is not produced, anuria. Peripheral nerve lesions cause loss of bladder tone. Diabetes and multiple sclerosis alter bladder function. Urinary retention is marked accumulation of urine in the bladder as a result of an inability to empty bladder. Nurse should assess the bladder for distention. Urinary infection may be caused by catheterization, poor perineal hygiene, local irritation, inadequate hand washing, failure to use proper method of washing from front to back after voiding or defection, frequent sexual intercourse, retention of urine. Dysuria is painful burning micturition.

Hematuria is blood tinged urine.

Urinary incontinence is—escape of urine from bladder. Leakage may be continuous or intermittent. Incontinence can be:

- Functional—unpredictable escape of urine with intact urinary and genital system
- Over flow—escape of 20–30 mL of urine after overdistension of bladder
- Reflex—escape as predictable intervals
- Stress—leakage due to increase in abdominal pressure
- Urge—escape after strong urge to void

It is common in older adults but may occur at any age.

Bladder training and use of indwelling catheter and condom drainage is used for incontinence of urine to prevent soiling.

Types and Collection of Urine Specimens

Types of sample for specimens:

- Random
- Midstream
- 24 hours collection
- Sterile sample for microscopic examination and culture
- Timed specimens.

Random

Collected during normal voiding, from indwelling catheter, from urinary diversion collection bag.

Assess voiding status of patient. Assess understanding of purpose, explain procedure to patient why, and how specimen is to be collected.

Give fluids half an hour before, if not contraindicated provide privacy by closing door or screening bed. Provide soap, water, washcloth to clean perineal area. Perform hand hygiene, wear gloves and assist non-ambulatory patient with bedpan. Change gloves (sterile) open wide mouth sterile specimen cup or bottle.

Clean with cotton ball urethra to anus separating labia with thumb and forefinger, pour sterile water, if needed. Ask client to void. After the stream is achieved collect 30–60 mL urine.

Remove container, make patient comfortable. Clean specimen bottle from outside, closing the container, place in plastic bag. Label specimen, fill laboratory form and send to the laboratory, wash hands. In case of male patient ask patient to clean glans penis with wet swab and collect midstream urine sample leaving first few milliliters of urine. Ask to collect 30–60 mL.

For simple urine analysis, a sample may not be sterile, only clean sample is needed. Patient can void in clean cup, urinal or bedpan, for sterile sample patient is catheterized and sample is collected in sterile container or culture bottle.

If patient is having indwelling catheter, sample can be collected through port by aseptic precaution. Clamp the tube 3 inches below the port, clean port with antiseptic swab, sterile needle on syringe and draw 3–5 mL of urine.

24 Hours Urine Collection

Collect urine for 24 hours. Indicate the time of starting, collect all urine voided in 24 hours.

Observation and Urine Testing

Equipment: Tray Containing

- Urine sample
- Urostrips
- Litmus paper
- Urinometer in container
- Spirit lamp
- Test tubes and test tube holder
- Matchbox, kidney tray, paper bag
- Benedict solution
- Acetic acid
- Nitric acid (if cold test for albumin)
- Measuring glass
- Dropper
- Gloves, hand washing articles
- Liquid ammonia, sulfur powder, tincher iodine, pour urine specimen in conical glass and observe (60–100 mL) (Fig. 10.13).

Color

Normally it is transparent, without sediments. Normally, color is pale yellow or amber. If output is less, urine is concentrated and color is dark. Abnormal colors are smoky, of blood, albumin, medication.

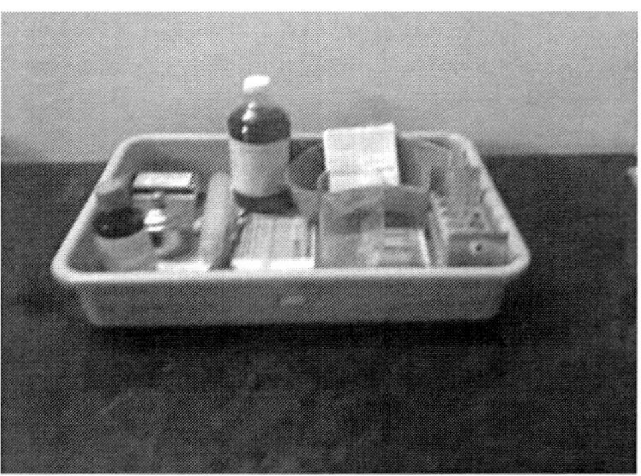

Fig. 10.13: Urine testing tray

Odor

Normally, it smells aromatic. Abnormal odors are fishy in infections, sweet or fruity when acetone is present in cases of diabetes mellitus and starving. Stale urine smells of ammonia.

Reaction

Dip the red and blue litmus paper. Normally the reaction is acidic, sometimes, alkaline turning red litmus blue.

Specific Gravity

Pour 100 mL of urine in container of urinometer. Place urinometer in container and read. Normally, specific gravity is 1.010–1.020. Dilute urine has less specific gravity, whereas if solutes are increased, specially protein and sugar, specific gravity will increase.

Test for Albumin

Hot Test

Fill the test tube 2/3 with urine. Light the spirit lamp and heat the upper part of the tube. Holding away from face. Observe for cloudy appearance by comparing the upper part with lower part of the urine in test tube. If clouds are observed, add 1–2 drops of acetic acid with the help of dropper.

If the clouds are due to phosphates they dissolve in acetic acid. If it is due to albumin, whiteness will remain. Albumin may be present in urine of patients with renal disease and congestive cardiac failure (CCF).

Cold Test

Take 1 mL of urine in test tube. Slide three to five drops of nitric acid along the test tube. If albumin is present due to coagulations of protein (albumin) there is formation of ring, white in color. The test is positive sliding of nitric acid is a procedure to be performed very carefully as the concentrated acid burns tissues.

Test for Sugar

Take 5 mL of benedicts solution. Heat the solution and see, if color changes. If color is changed throw the solution, do not use as it is not fresh. Take fresh solution, heat it the color should remain as it is (blue). Add 8 drops of urine in heated urine. Again heat the solution. Observe the color–

Blue—No sugar present
Green—0. 5% sugar present +
Yellow—01% sugar present ++
Orange—1. 5% sugar present +++
Brick red—2% and above ++++

Acetone Test

Rothera's Test

Take one teaspoon crystals of ammonium sulfate in test tube. Add 15 drops of urine and one crystal of sodium nitroprusside.

Shake the test tube after putting cork. Add liquor ammonia trickling through sides. Read the results immediately. Purple color ring is formed at the junction. In modern method, dipping the urostrip the changes in color indicate presence of sugar, albumin, acetone, and blood.

The strip can be used to detect presence of these.

Test for Bile Salts

Hay's Test

Take half test tube full of urine. Sprinkle sulfur powder on surface, if powder sinks, it indicates presence of bile salts.

Test for Bile Pigments

Smith's test fill 3/4 test tube with urine, form a layer by sliding iodine drops gently from the sides of the test tube. If green ring at the junction is formed, it indicates presence of bile pigments.

Discard urine, wash hands clean, replace articles and wash hands.

Facilitating Urine Elimination

Providing Privacy

The degree of privacy needed for urination varies. Consider cultural, social and gender habits. Standing, sitting, squatting positions may help in urination.

Anxiety and emotional stress may cause urgency and frequency and prevent complete emptying. Increase the intake of fluid to increase output. Tea, coffee, cold drinks increase urine formation. Alcohol inhibits antidiuretic hormone (ADH). Diuresis takes place. If urinary retention occurs to facilitate urination offer bedpan, pour hot and cold water alternately on genitals. Let the patient hear the noise from tap water. Place hot water bottle on suprapubic region. Provide privacy. Release bladder with catheterization if all measures fail. Catheterization should be performed with all aseptic precautions.

Condom Drainage

It is suitable for comatose or incontinent patient. It is soft, pliable, rubber sheath that slips over penis. It may be used continuously or at night.

Condom catheter can be secured in place by these methods:

- Use of strip of elastic tape or rubber encircling the top of the condom
- Self-adhesive condom sheath
- Inflatable ring within the condom to secure. While securing, it is must that there is no obstruction to blood flow to penis. Sticking plaster or standard adhesive tape should never be used because it does not expand with change in penis size and is painful to remove. Elastic tape applied in a spiral manner.

Attach end of the condom to plastic drainage tubing that is attached to side of the bed or strapped to the patients leg. If it is made from opaque material it should be removed daily to check for skin irritation. Tubing must be checked for patency.

PERINEAL CARE

Purpose

- As a part of bed bath
- Clients with risk of infection in cases of perineal surgery, parturition, urinary catheters, menstruation, rectal and genital surgery.

Equipment

Mackintosh and draw sheet, bath towel, bedpan. Warm water in basin, soap dish and soap swabs, toilet tissue, wash cloths, and gloves.

Procedure

Screen the patient and provide privacy. Explain the procedure and assess the knowledge, prepare tray and take to bedside. Raise bed to comfortable height. Lower side rails, place mackintosh, draw sheet, underneath and bath towel in length on side. Cover patient with bath blanket. Wear gloves. Clean buttocks and anus, wash hip front to back. Keep cotton pad, if needed. Pour water on genitals or swab front to back. Dry area, change gloves, if soiled. Apply perineal pad, if needed. Remove mackintosh and draw sheet make patient comfortable, wash hands.

For females, use wet swabs to clean labia majora, minora and urethra, vestibule. Two swabs for labia majora from above downwards. Open labia majora and clean labia minora with two swabs from above downwards and one swab centrally for clitoris and vestibule.

CATHETERIZATION

Catheterization of bladder is introducing rubber or plastic catheter through urethra into the urinary bladder.

Types: Intermittent catheterization, indwelling or self-retaining catheters.

Straight catheter for single use has small opening on lumen at 1/2 inch distance from tip French number 8–10 for adults and 4–6 for children (Fig. 10.14).

Indwelling catheter or Foley's catheter (Fig. 10.15) has small inflatable balloon that encircles catheter at the tip with two to three lumens. Balloon can be inflated with 10 mL of saline or air to retain the catheter after introducing in bladder and deflated before removing the catheter from bladder—polythene catheter is less traumatic and used for male patients and is with curved tip. Indwelling catheter can be placed for short-term or long-term.

Intermittent catheter can be repeated as necessary, but there is risk of injury and infection (Fig 10.16). Catheter is introduced for single use till bladder is empty and removed at once. Check the doctor's order for catheterization.

Assess bladder. Check patient's gender and age, mobility and limitations. Wash hands. Inspect perineum for rash, drainage, odor, and allergies.

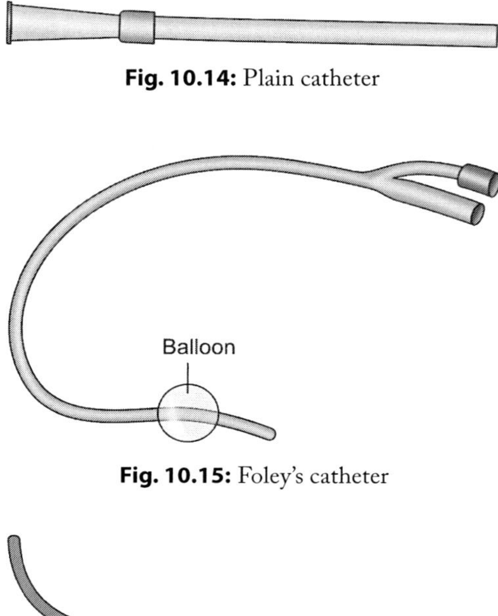

Fig. 10.14: Plain catheter

Fig. 10.15: Foley's catheter

Fig. 10.16: Metal catheter

Assess patient's knowledge for purpose of procedure, explain the procedure to patient, arrange for assistance, if required. Wash hands, screen the patient or close door, raise bed to appropriate height, clear the bedside table. Stand one side of bed usually right place equipment. Raise side rail on opposite side and lower down on working side.

Place mackintosh under the buttocks. Position the patient.

Drape the patient. Cover extremities with sheet exposing genitalia or put leggings and hole towel. Wear disposable gloves. Wash perineal area with soap and water as needed, discard gloves. Wash hands, arrange for proper light. Wear sterile gloves, organize supplies on sterile field by opening sterile package containing catheter, lubricant (arrange in a sterile tray a catheter, sterile bowl with savlon swabs, sterile container to collect specimen, sterile lubricant in bottle).

Lubricate catheter 2.5–5 cm for females and 12.5–17.7 cm for males.

Place hole towel (Sterile) after gloving without touching other parts (unsterile objects). Clean labial folds using antiseptic swabs using one swab for one area wiping from front to back from clitoris towards anus.

Pick-up catheter with gloved hand, 3–4 inches away from the tip and hold catheter loosely coiled in hand or grasp the catheter in forceps. Ask patient to bear down as it for voiding and insert catheter 2–3 inches till urine comes.

CARE OF URINARY DRAINAGE

When indwelling catheter is placed in bladder, it is secured to inner thigh with strip of tape or velcro strap. It is placed slack to allow movement of thigh and prevent tension on catheter. It also reduces pressure on urethra and reduces injury. In males, secure tubing on top of the thigh or lower abdomen. Attach end of retention catheter to collecting tube of drainage tube.

Make sure there are no obstructions in tubing, coiling of tube, fasten to the bottom sheet with clip or rubber band and safety pin. Keep drainage bag below the level of bladder. Attach bag to bed frame. Do not place on side rails.

To maintain the patency of indwelling catheter, it is required sometimes to flush or irrigate to clear blood, pus, or sediments which collect sometimes within the tube. Sterile solution ordered is pushed for infection antiseptic or antibiotic bladder irrigation may be ordered. Sterile aseptic technique is used.

Do not allow spigot to touch a contaminated surface. Use sterile technique when collecting urine sample. If tube becomes disconnected, do not touch end of tube or catheter wipe with antiseptic before reconnecting. Use separate receptacle to measure output to prevent cross infection. Prevent pulling reflux of urinary bladder. If raising is required during transport, clamp the tube. Before exercise or ambulation, drain all urine from the tubing to drainage bag. Avoid prolonged kinking or clamping tube encourage fluid intake. Remove catheter as soon as clinically warranted. Perform routine perineal care. Report and record type of catheter, size, inserted and amount of fluid used to inflate balloon, characteristics of urine, reason for catheterization, specimen collected, patient's response to procedure and teaching. Initiate intake output chart. If no urine is produced within an hour, report immediately to physician. Client's at home may use leg bag during day and large volume bag during night.

CARE OF URINARY DIVERSIONS

Urinary diversions—a urinary stoma to divert the flow of urine from the kidneys directly to the abdominal surface is created.

It may be temporary or permanent.

It is created in cases of cancer bladder, trauma, radiation injury, fistula and cystitis.

Types

Ileal Loop or Conduit (Fig. 10.17)

It is separating a loop of intestinal ileum with its blood supply intact. The ureters are implanted into isolated segment of ileum. The remaining ileum is reconnected to the rest of the digestive tract. Client wears stomal pouch continuously.

Continent Urinary Diversion

Ureterostomy

End of one or both ureters is brought to abdominal surface (Figs 10.18A to D).

Transureteroureterostomy

Connects the ureters and one is brought out through abdominal wall.

Nephrostomy Tube is Placed in Renal Pelvis

When incontinence of urine is present stomal pouch is worn continuously as there is no sphincter.

Local irritation of skin may be caused due to long contact with urine.

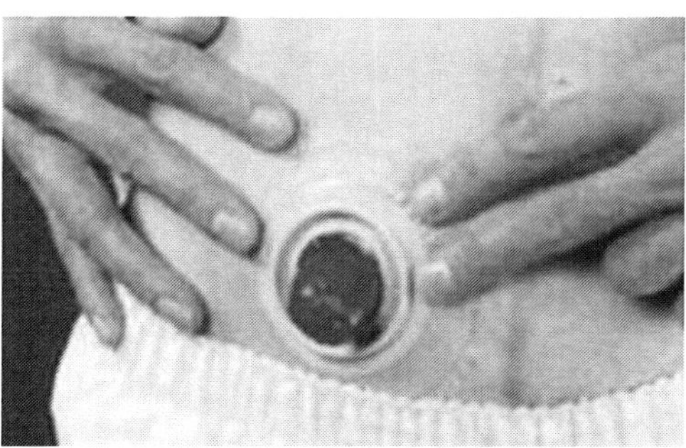

Fig. 10.17: Ileal conduit

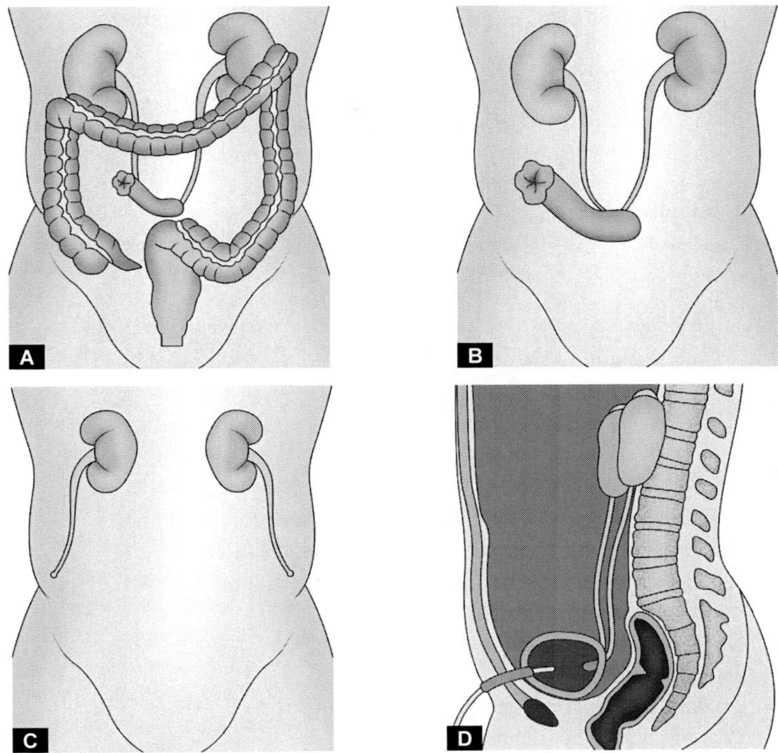

Fig. 10.18A to D: Types of urinary diversions. (A)Ileal loop; (B) Transureterostomy; (C) Double ureterostomy; (D) Continent urinary diversion

It creates problem of body image. Wearing of artificial device to collect urine is required. It does not obstruct activities of daily living.

Pouch is constructed to provide urinary storage in leakproof puller. Portion of ileum connected to abdominal wall acts as continent nipple, and requires intermittent catheterization. Complications may occur like infection, hydronephrosis, if outflow is obstructed.

BLADDER IRRIGATION

It is washing out bladder cavity with a stream of lotion or water (Table 10.8).

Table 10.8: Equipment and types of bladder irrigation

Types of irrigation		*Equipment*
Continuous method	-	Tray containing sterile irrigation set, bulb syringe or 60 mL syringe, sterile basin, mackintosh, sterile solution in a container, antiseptic swabs. Sterile gloves, tape or elastic band, sheet or bath blanket
Open method		
Closed method	-	Sterile irrigation solution at room temperature. Irrigation tubing and clamp IV Pole, antiseptic swabs. Y connection sheet or bath blanket
Closed intermittent method	-	Sterile irrigation solution at room temperature. Sterile graduated container, sterile syringe 30–50 mL, sterile 19–22 gauge needle, antiseptics swab. Clamp for catheter—sheet or bath blanket

Procedure

- See doctor's order for type of irrigations, solution
- Observe color of urine, presence of mucus, sedimentations
- See catheter in place, the type—triple lumen, double lumen
- Look for patency of tube
- Observe amount of urine in drainage bag
- Empty the bag, if full
- Explain the procedure to patient and purpose
- Wash hands, wear clean gloves
- Provide privacy
- Cover patient with one sheet (upper torso)
- Observe bladder for distention
- Give supine or dorsal recumbent position
- Prepare sterile solution ordered
- Draw sterile solution into syringe
- Clamp port with antiseptic solution
- Clean port with antiseptic solution
- Insert needle through port at 30° angle towards bladder
- Withdraw syringe, remove clamp and allow solution to drain into drainage bag or as per order, retain the fluid for 20 minutes and then release clamp.

Closed Continuous Irrigation

Using aseptic technique insert tip of sterile irrigation tubing into bag of sterile irrigation solution. Close clamp on tubing and hang bag of solution on IV stand. Open clamp, allow solution to flow, close clamp.

Wipe irrigation port of triple lumen catheter or attaching sterile Y connection to double lumen catheter then attach to irrigation tubing clamp tubing on drainage and open clamp on irrigation tubing, allow 100 mL to enter the bladder and close irrigation clamp, open drainage tubing clamp keep 20 minutes solution in bladder, if ordered.

If continuous drainage calculate drip rate and adjust clamp on irrigation tubing confirm patency of tubing and keep open clamp drainage tubing and check volume of drainage in drainage bag (Fig. 10.19).

Open Irrigation

- Establish sterile field
- Pour required sterile irrigation solution in sterile container from large container
- Wear sterile gloves
- Place mackintosh or waterproof drape under catheter
- Aspirate 30 mL solution in syringe
- Disconnect catheter from tubing
- Allow urine from catheter to flow into basin, kidney tray cover drainage tube with cap. Secure tubing

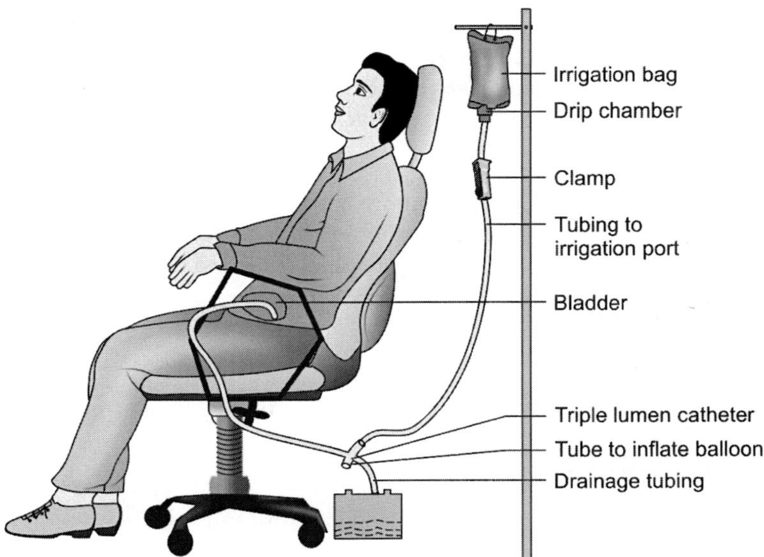

Fig. 10.19: Closed continuous bladder irrigation

- Insert tip of syringe into catheter. Instill solution, withdraw syringe, lower catheter, allow solution to drain in basin
- Repeat instilling solution till clear solution returns
- If solution does not return, change patient's position still if solution does not return gently, aspirate
- After irrigation is complete, connect drainage tube to catheter clearing end
- Secure catheter and tubing
- Give comfortable position
- Lower the bed and put side rails
- Dispose contaminated supplies, remove gloves, wash hands
- Calculate, observe and check the results.

BOWEL ELIMINATION

Normally the rectum is empty. When the fecal mass or gas moves into rectum to distend its walls, defecation begins.

Process involves involuntary and voluntary control. As the rectum distends, sensory impulse stimulates to relax sphincters. External and internal sphincters relax. Adults and toilet trained children can voluntarily control external sphincter. Pressure can be increased by increasing intra-abdominal pressure or a valsalva maneuver.

Valsalva maneuver is voluntary contraction of abdominal muscles during forced expiration with closed glottis (holding breath).

Constipation

Decrease in frequency of bowel movement accompanied by prolonged and difficult passing of hard, dry stools. Efforts to pass stools can cause problem of giving away sutures, hypertension, elevated intraocular pressure and increased intracranial pressure, fecal impaction.

Diarrhea

Increase in number of stools and passage of unformed liquid stools.

Fecal Incontinence

Inability to control passage of feces and gas from anus.

Flatulence : Accumulation of gas in intestines.

Hemorrhoids : Dilated, engorged veins in rectum.

Composition and Characteristics of Feces (Table 10.9)

Composition

Undigested food, dead bacteria, fat, bile pigments, cells lining intestinal wall, mucus, and water.

Observation

Observe for amount, color, and consistency. Look for abnormal constituents like blood, mucus, fat, pus, foreign bodies, worms, abnormal color may be white, black tarry, reddish. Black color may be due to oral iron therapy, intestinal bleeding, pale in jaundice.

Consistency

Liquid, watery, semisolid, diarrhea, dysentery, cholera, food poisoning presence of mucus and blood in dysentery, inflammations, frothy in malabsorption syndrome, enteritis, Prune's disease.

Factors Affecting Bowel Elimination

Age

Infant has small stomach and less enzymes for digestion. Complex starch is poorly tolerated. Rapid peristalsis push food fast. Infant is unable to control as less sphincter control exists.

Table 10.9: Characteristics of feces

Characteristic	*Normal*	*Abnormal*
1. Color	Infant—yellow Adult—brown	White, clay, black, red, pale, mucus
2. Odor	Pungent affected by food type	Noxious
3. Consistency	Soft, well-formed	Liquid, hard
4. Frequency	Infants—4–6	6 or more
	Adults—1–3	Once in 2–3 days
5. Amount	150 g/day	
6. Shape	Resembles diameter of rectum	

Older adults loose muscle tone in perineal region, and anal sphincter. Incontinence may be present, irregular bowel movements and constipation.

Diet

Fiber—undigestable food residual diet provides bulk of fecal matter, grains, fruits, vegetables absorb water, increases stool mass. Defecation reflex occurs. Lactose containing foods may create distention.

Fluid Intake

Fluid liquifies intestinal contents. Reduced fluid intake slows passage of food. Increased intakes of milk slow peristalsis.

Physical Activity

It promotes peristalsis. Immobilization depresses peristalsis. Weak pelvic, floor muscles, abdominal muscles impaired intra-abdominal pressure and there is risk of constipation.

Psychological Factors

In problem, fear, anxiety, anger peristalsis is increased. Stress, depression reduces peristalsis resulting in constipation.
Ulcerative colitis, peptic ulcer can result due to stress.

Personal Habits

Using own toilet facility is effective and convenient. Busy work schedule may prevent to respond to urge to defecate.

Lack of privacy in hospital, sharing of toilet facilities, use of bed pan, sights sounds and odors associated with sharing toilet may be embarrassing to patients.

Position during defecation—squatting, exerting intra-abdominal pressure, contracting thigh muscles, helps in defection.

Pain—to avoid pain from hemorrhoids, surgery, fistula person tries to avoid defection.

Pregnancy—constipation may occur in 3rd trimester.

Surgery and anesthesia—GA affects peristalsis.

Medications promoting defecation and controlling diarrheas medicines affect peristalsis movements.

Alterations in Bowel Elimination

Constipation

In frequent bowel movements, difficult evacuation of feces, inability to defecate at will, hard feces, straining at the time of defecation. Passage of dry, hard stool.

Impaction

Fecal impaction results from unrelieved constipation. Hard feces are collected and wedged in rectum and cannot be expelled. Unconscious patients, confused or debilitated patients may suffer from impaction.

Diarrhea

Increase in number of stools. Passing of liquid, unformed stools. Diseases affecting digestion, absorption may result in diarrhea. Feces are watery and uncontrolled, large to defecate.

Fecal incontinence: Inability to control passage of feces and gas from anus. It can harm body image. Impaired anal sphincter can cause incontinence.

Flatulence: It is cause of distention of abdomen pain and cramping. Belching and passing of gases reduces distention.

Hemorrhoids: Veins in the rectal mucosa are dilated and engorged.

Collection of Specimen (Feces)

Nurse is directly responsible for ensuring.

- Obtaining accurate specimen
- Correct labeling
- Appropriate container
- Transportation to laboratory on time.

Instruct patient how to collect feces in container. To avoid mixing of water or urine ask patient to defecate in clean, dry bedpan or special container placed under the toilet seat.

For occult blood and culture, small amount of specimen is needed.

Wash hands, wear gloves, with wooden spatula collect about inch of formed stool or 15–30 mL of liquid diarrhea stool. Label correctly and seal tightly, wash hands, remove gloves. Fill laboratory form and send to laboratory.

Observation (Table 10.10)

Table 10.10: Observation of specimen (feces)

S. No	*Observation*	*Normal*	*Abnormal*
1.	Color	Infant—yellow	White, clay, black, red, pale with mucus
2.	Odor	Pungent affected by food type	Blood, mucus noxious change
3.	Consistency	Soft, formed	Liquid, hard
4.	Frequency	Infant—4–6 times Adult—2–3 times	> 6 times < Once > 3 times/day < 1 in week
5.	Amount	Adult 150 g/day diameter of rectum	
6.	Constituents	Undigested food, dead bacteria, bile pigment, fat, water, intestinal muscle cells	Blood, pus, foreign bodies mucus, worms, excess fat

Giving Bedpan and Removing Bedpan

Bedridden patients or clients restricted to bed must use bedpans for defection. For women, passing of urine and stool bedpan is required. Men use bedpan for defecation. Bedpan made-up of metal, enamel, plastic material has curved smooth upper end and sharp edged lower end and it is 5 cm deep.

Upper end fits under buttocks and lower end under thighs.

Before giving it is to be warmed with hot water and then dried.

Always avoid strain and discomfort of patient sitting or lying on bedpan. Never leave him or her alone and go. Make bed flat when giving bedpan and raise the head to 30° after giving it. Maintain privacy. Provide cleaning papers and call bell. Remove gently and putting on gloves clean anal and perineal area.

Cleaning Patients after Giving Bedpan and Cleaning Bedpans and Urinals

Equipment

Tray containing large swabs in bowl or pieces of cloth in bowl. Warm water in pint measure.

Gloves or dissecting forceps, kidney tray, soap swabs.

Keep clean bedpan under the buttocks after removing used bedpan and cover it.

Pour warm water over perineum and anal area.

Clean from perineum to anus using one wet swab or piece of cloth at a time in forceps or gloved hand. Do not bring back the swab in reverse direction. Use soap swabs and again clean with wet swabs. Pour water again, if needed. Dry with dry piece of cloth or paper towel.

Remove bedpan, remove gloves. Give back care and comfortable position. Change the draw sheet, if required.

Observe stool. Empty bedpan in toilet. A spray faucet attached to toilet allows rinsing of bedpan thoroughly. Put 50 mL of diluted disinfectant after washing. Use same bedpan for same patient. Offer bedpan often before he/she soils clothes.

ENEMA

Enema is the instillation of a solution into the rectum and sigmoid colon.

Purpose

- To promote defecation by stimulating peristalsis
- To break the fecal mass, stretch rectal wall
- To introduce drug to effect on local mucosa
- To empty the bowel before diagnostic test surgery, child birth
- To begin program of bowel training.

Types

- Cleaning enema—tap water, normal saline, soap solution, low volume hypertonic saline
- Carminative
- Return flow enema
- Medicated enema.

Cleansing Enema

Large amounts of water, saline stimulate peristalsis, irritate colonic mucus and promote complete evacuation of bowel.

Amount of solution for adults 750–1000 mL, adolescent 500–750 mL, children 300–500 mL, infants 150–250 mL, toddler 250–350 mL. For infants and toddlers only normal saline is to be used as other solutions may create fluid imbalance.

Tap water is hypotonic, exerts low osmotic pressure than fluid in intestinal space, fluid escaping to these spaces after absorption from colon. Repeated water toxication or circulatory overload may occur, if large amounts of water are absorbed.

Normal saline is safe as it is physiological solution. It exerts same osmotic pressure as interstitial fluids. Infused saline stimulates peristalsis. It does not create danger of excess fluid absorption. Prepare saline, if not available—mix 500 mL water and 1 tablespoon table salt (Nacl).

General Principles of Administrations

Nurse administers enema in commercially packed, disposable units or with reusable equipment prepared before use.

- Explaining procedure, giving position and the precautions to be taken are to be explained before administering enema
- Enema is given till clear fluid comes out and contain no fecal matter
- See that no air enters while giving enema
- Hold enema can 18" above bed level and ask the patient to take deep breaths
- Pinch the tube before solution is finished and remove catheter
- Apply vaseline before inserting catheter into anus
- If prepacked disposable container is used remove plastic cap from rectal tip. Tip is already lubricated but more jelly can be applied
- Gently separate buttocks. Instruct patient to breathe out
- Insert tip of bottle in to rectum. Adult 3"–4" and child 2"–3" infant 1"
- Squeeze bottle until all solution enters rectum and colon. Ask to retain for five minutes.

Administration of Different Enemas (Table 10.11)

Table 10.11: Administration of different enemes

Returned enemas	*Retained enemas*
500–1000 mL	30–200 mL
Add warm solution to enema bag	1. Starch and mucilage enema
Raise container, release clamp	2. Black tea or coffee
Allow solution to flow, reclamp tubing	3. Paraldehyde 2 mL, diluted in water

Contd...

Contd...

Returned enemas	*Retained enemas*
Lubricate 2"–4" of tip. Separate buttocks. Instruct patient to breathe out. Insert rectal tube tip into rectum. 3"–4". Hold tube in rectum till fluid is instilled. Open clamp and allow solution to enter slowly hold container at hip level. Raise height to 12"–18" clamp tubing when all solution is instilled. Place toilet tissue around tube and gently withdraw rectal tube. Ask patient to retain solution as long as possible. Discard enema cane and tubing in proper receptacles. Assist client to bathroom or help on bedpan. Observe stool passed. Record the enema and result	4. Ice water
	It is given after cleansing enema
	It is given by drip method
	Clip is attached to the rubber tubing and glass connection and a rectal catheter
	Drip can be given with funnel or syringe barrel
	Empty infusion bottle attaching a tube and connection with clip

BOWEL WASH OR COLONIC IRRIGATION

Bowel wash is washing out off bowel contents. It is also called as colonic lavage, irrigation or enteroclysis.

Definition

Introduction of large volume of fluid into large intestine in a steady stream under low pressure in order to wash out material accumulated above the rectum and to lavage the intestinal wall.

Purpose

- To clean bowel of feces, gas, excess mucus, bacterias, barium and toxins
- To prepare colon for specific surgical and diagnostic procedures
- To reduce temperature in hyperpyrexia and heat stroke
- To supply fluid and electrolytes that are absorbed from intestines
- To stimulate peristalsis

- To reduce inflammation
- To keep individual clean in fecal incontinence.

Contraindications

Bleeding hemorrhoids, chronic diarrhea, rectal surgeries, infection, intestinal obstruction, rectal polyps, massive colon carcinoma, anal skin lesions.

Solutions Used

Plain water, cold water, normal saline, 1% sodium bicarbonate, Condy's lotion. 005%, boric lotion 1%, aluminum 1%.

Amount of Solution Used

About 2–3 liters, at temperature of 104–106°F for cleansing purpose, 80–90°F for reducing temperature.

Prerequisites

- Cleansing enema before one hour
- Empty bladder.

Equipment

A tray containing funnel and rectal tube, or Y connection tubing and rectal catheter, vaseline, swabs, rag pieces, kidney tray, mackintosh, solution in jug, pint measure, bucket, bedpan, perineal toilet tray, plastic apron and disposable gloves.

Procedure

- Check the physician's order
- See any specific instructions
- Explain the procedure and purpose to the patient
- Position the patient in left lateral position bringing at the edge of the bed
- Place mackintosh and draw sheet underneath, folding top linen at the foot end and covering the patient with single sheet
- Wash hands, apply gloves, attach tubing and rectal tube
- Check temperature of fluid, pour solution and check for leakage

- Lubricate the catheter 4 inches from the tip, fill funnel with solution, allow the air to escape by flowing the solution in kidney tray
- Pinch the tube or clamp, maintaining left lateral position insert catheter tip 4 inches separating buttocks with other hand and ask patient to exhale deep breath
- Release clamp or pinch, lower the funnel to allow the gas to escape, then raise the funnel and allow fluid to run in
- Continue pouring more fluid into funnel before it is empty. Pour 200–300 mL fluid and then invert the funnel into bucket
- Repeat pouring of fluid holding funnel upright above buttocks
- Repeat procedure till clear fluid comes out
- Ask patient if he comfortable or not during procedure
- Gently remove the rectal tube with rag piece and discard
- Wipe catheter and keep in kidney tray
- Assist patient for toilet, give perineal care, if needed
- Wipe and dry buttocks, remove mackintosh and draw sheet, change sheet, if soiled.
- Assist for lying down comfortably, cover patient, put on fan, remove screen, if used
- Dispose gloves, wash and disinfect tubing and funnel, wash hands and replace articles
- Record the result, time of procedure and condition of patient.

SITZ BATH

Provides warmth to perineal area and anus. Gives relief from pain and reduces swelling.

Equipment

Large basin, hot and cold water, Condy's lotion or betadine solution, bath thermometer, towel and mackintosh.

Procedure

- Check physician's order
- Explain the procedure to the patient
- Assess the patient's condition
- Patient may sit in water filled basin in bathroom or on bed
- Place mackintosh and draw sheet over bed folding top clothes to foot end of the bed

- Mix hot and cold water half basin full. Check temperature of water with bath thermometer or at the inner aspect of forearm. Temperature should be 105–110° F. Add few drops of Condy's lotion or betadine to water
- Remove dressing or perineal pad, if applied
- Make the patient to sit on basin dipping anal and perineal area
- Patient can sit on stool or potty chair
- Ask the patient to sit for 20 minutes
- Change water, if becomes cold
- Ask the patient to getout of basin
- Dry the area, remove mackintosh and draw sheet
- Apply pad or dressing, if needed
- Make the patient comfortable, wash hands, clean and replace articles
- Chart the treatment, time and result.

CARE OF OSTOMIES

Ostomies require pouch to collect feces. Effective pouching system protects the skin, contains feces and it is odor proof and concealable.

It consists of pouch and skin barrier. Pouches are disposable or reusable, in one piece or two pieces. Skin barriers include wafers, pastes, powders or liquid film. It is applied to the skin around stoma. Pouch is changed when there is little drainage from ostomy, before meals and bedtime.

Equipment

Pouch system, clamp, gloves, deodorant, gauze or washcloths, towel or disposable waterproof barrier, basin with warm water, scissors, pen and stethoscope.

Procedure

- Auscultate for bowel sounds
- Observe pouch for leakage and length of time in place
- Observe stoma for color, swelling, trauma, and healing
- Normally it is moist, reddish pink or like a bud
- Remove skin barrier and pouch after observing effluence from stoma
- Assess skin around stoma
- Explain procedure to client, talk to him, answer his queries
- Bring equipment near to bed
- Drape the client
- Place towel underneath after washing hands and gloving

- Remove pouch and skin barrier gently
- Clean peristomal skin gently with warm water with gauze or washcloth. Do not scrub
- Dry completely by patting with gauze or towel, measure stoma.
- In cut-to-fit pouch, cut 1/6 or 1/8 inch larger than stoma before removing pack
- With ileostomy apply thin circle of barrier paste around opening in pouch and allow it to dry
- Apply skin barrier and pouch (Fig. 10.20). If crease is seen, fill it with barrier paste and let it dry
- Gently tug on pouch in downward direction after applying pouch and a fingertip pressure.

PASSING OF FLATUS TUBE

Flatus tube is passed into rectum to pass flatus and relieve distention of abdomen.

Equipment

A tray containing mackintosh, towel, flatus tube, bowl of water, rag pieces, vaseline, kidney tray.

Procedure

- Collect equipment and keep on the stool near patients foot end
- Explain the procedure to patient
- Close the room or screen the bed. Measure abdominal girth

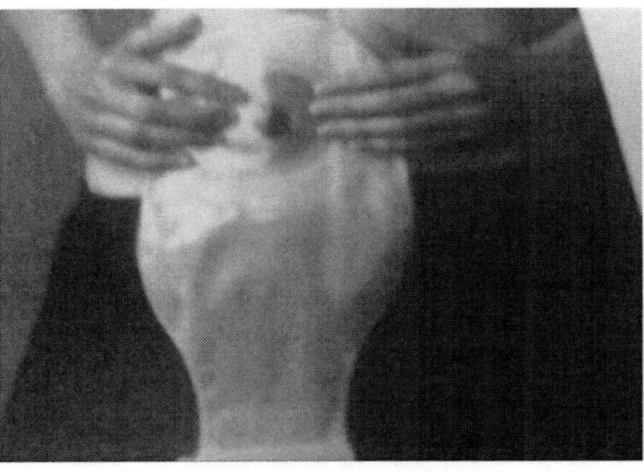

Fig. 10.20: Colostomy pouch

- Put off the fan. Give left lateral position to patient
- Place mackintosh and towel under the buttocks removing top sheet and blanket to foot of the bed
- Lubricate the flatus tube with vaseline 3–4 inches
- Insert the flatus tube through anal opening into rectum (Fig. 10.21)
- Place the distal end of the tube in water filled kidney tray. Bubble will be seen on escape of gas
- Keep the tube in place for sometime and observe
- Measure abdominal girth. Remove tube slowly and wrap in rag piece
- Mark the result
- Remove mackintosh and towel
- Comfort the patient
- Wash hands, replace the articles after washing and sterilizing.

MOBILITY AND IMMOBILITY

Principles of Body Mechanics

Body mechanics is the efficient use of the body as a machine and as a means of locomotion. It consists of posture, balance and movements.

Posture

Position in which the various parts of the body are held while sitting, standing, lying down and walking.

Balance

Equilibrium.

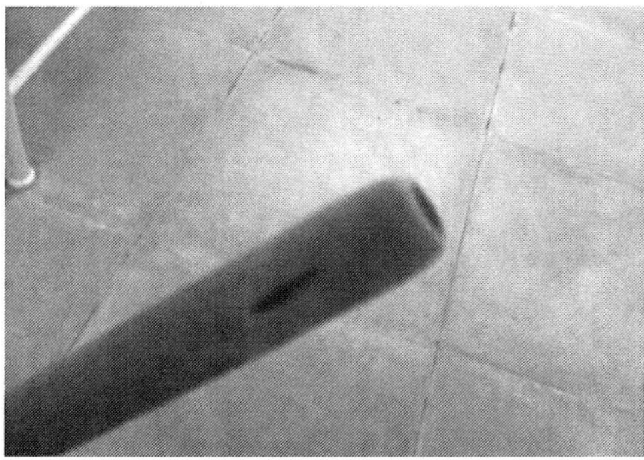

Fig. 10.21: Flatus tube

Movements

Flexion, extension, adduction, abduction, medial rotation or internal rotation, lateral or external rotation, circumduction, pronation, and supination.

Nervous system, muscles, tendons, bones, joints are involved in maintaining posture, balance and movements.

Body mechanics is coordinated efforts of musculoskeletal and nervous system to maintain balance, posture and body alignment while lifting, moving, performing activities of daily living.

Principles

- Object is stable when center of gravity is close to its base and line of gravity passing in the center or near to center
- Longest and strongest muscles should be used for energy
- Immobility can lead to contractures
- Correct posture when standing, head is erect and in midline, shoulders and hips are parallel and straight, spinal curves are reverse S pattern, abdomen, knees and ankles are slightly flexed, arms hang comfortably on sides, feet are placed slightly apart to achieve base of support. Toes are pointed forward, center of gravity is in midline, line of gravity is from middle of forehead to midpoint between feet
- When sitting head is erect, neck and vertebral column are straight, body weight is evenly distributed on buttocks and thighs
- When lying in lateral position, vertebral column is straight and without observable curves.

Lifting Heavy Objects

When lifting heavy objects, tighten abdominal muscles, and tuck pelvis, bend at knees, keep weight to be lifted as close to body as possible. Maintain trunk erect and knees bent, avoid twisting. Best height to lift is 2 feet off the ground. To reach the object overhead, use safe stable stool or ladder, avoid standing on tiptoe, stand close to shelf, transfer weight of object from shelf to arms and over the base of support.

Maintaining Normal Body Alignment and Mobility

Body alignment: It is relationship of one body part to another along a horizontal or vertical line. Correct alignment reduces muscle strain. Body balance is achieved when relatively lower center of gravity is balanced over a wide stable base of support. Body balance is enhanced by posture. Posture means maintaining optimal body position which requires least muscular work and favors function. Coordinated body movements involve skeletal, muscular and nervous system. Joint, ligaments, bones, tendons, skeletal muscles support the body, move and give strength. Body contour and form depends on muscles.

Gravity pulls on parts of the body all the time. Muscles exert pull on opposite direction.

Good posture places less strain on muscles and prevents fatigue. Semicircular canals, cerebellum are responsible in maintaining balance of the body. Proprioception is awareness of the position of the body and its parts. Proprioceptors monitor muscle activity and body position. Voluntary area located in cerebral cortex controls muscle movements. Patient's body alignment is to be maintained in different positions.

In supine position, client rests on back, needs foot support. In Fowler's position, head is elevated 45–60° and knees are slightly flexed, support to maintain normal spinal curves. In prone position, turn head to one side, client lies on abdomen with support of pillow under head. Wedge can be placed under chest or arms flexed overhead, pillow under lower leg for relaxation or dorsiflexion of ankle over end of the mattress.

In lateral positions, client is supported on left or right side with opposite arm, thigh, knee flexed and resting on bed, pillow to support at the back.

Factors Affecting Body Alignment and Mobility

- **Developmental changes:** Newborn's body is flexible and lacks body curves. As the child grows, stability increases. Thoracic spine straightens. Standing and walking is possible. Within 3–15 years musculoskeletal system grows and develops. Aging limits musculoskeletal activities
- **Postural abnormalities:** Scoliosis, kyphosis, lordosis may result from faulty posture
- **Abnormalities in bone formation:** Rickets, congenital deformities like genu valgum, genu varum, other deformities of the spine and limbs may affect body alignment, movement and self-image
- **Damage to central nervous system:** Damage to cerebral cortex, cerebellum will result in restriction or loss of movements
- **Trauma to musculoskeletal system:** Fracture, dislocation, sprain, wounds, torsion restricts client's body movements.

Hazards Associated with Immobility

- **Contracture:** Joints that are not moved periodically can develop contracture. Permanent shortening of muscle followed by shortening of ligaments and tendons. Joint may become fixed in one position and client loses normal use of joint
- **Skin breakdown:** Peripheral blood flow may be affected especially in clients with diabetes, obesity, vascular disease and pressure may create skin breakdown
- **Venous thrombosis:** Peripheral venous flow especially in lower limbs may be affected, if not moved and venous congestion may result in venous thrombosis
- **Thrombophlebitis:** Stagnation of venous blood in veins of lower limb may lead to inflammation
- **Foot drop:** Client without support to feet especially with hemiplegia, paraplegia, unconsciousness may develop foot drop, if proper support and exercise is not given
- **Disturbed body image:** Contractures, deformities, loss of body part may disturb body image
- **Activity intolerance:** Muscle weakness, fatigue, paralysis, fractures and other deformities result in activity intolerance
- **Risk for injury:** Problems of balance, activity intolerance and others may cause risk for injury.

Nursing Diagnosis and Interventions

- Activity intolerance
- Impaired physical mobility related to pain in joint
- Risk for disuse syndrome
- Risk for impaired skin integrity.

Interventions

- Health promotion activities
  - Education—Lifting, self-care, exercise
  - Prevention
  - Early detection.
- Acute care based interventions—positioning, transferring
- Adequate exchange of respiratory gases
- Use of Ambu bag in unconscious patient
- Nasotracheal and orotracheal suctioning

- Assist client to move, maintain muscle tone
- Discourage Valsalva maneuver
- Ask client to breathe on getting up
- Leg exercises
- Deep breathing exercises, coughing exercises
- Encourage fluids, nutrient supplements
- Change of position, sleeves/stockings
- Chest physiotherapy
- Maintaining patent airway, proper positioning
- 2000–3000 mL intake
- Indwelling catheter for incontinence
- Motivate for ADL
- Use of foot board, trochanter roll, trapezius bar.

OXYGENATION

Review of Cardiovascular and Respiratory Physiology

Oxygen is required by all the cells of the body. Cardiac and respiratory systems provide it (Fig. 10.22). Blood is oxygenated through process of ventilation.

Perfusion and transport of gases (Fig. 10.23). Neural and chemical regulators control the rate and depth of respiration in response to changing oxygen demands. Blood from lower part of the body returns to right auricle of the heart via inferior vena cava and via superior vena cava from upper part of body. It is pushed into respiratory system via pulmonary artery and in lungs it combines with oxygen and gives off carbon dioxide. Blood then returns via four pulmonary veins to left auricle of the heart and to left ventricle, which contracts to pump it into aorta, systemic circulation. Cardiac output, cardiac index, stroke volume, preload and afterload are the factors responsible for blood flow regulation. Electrical impulse from sinoatrial (SA) node to heart muscles make rhythmic contractions of heart muscles. Ventilation is process of moving gases into and out of lungs. Breathing is an effort required for expanding and contracting lungs. Inspiration is active process and expiration is passive process. Diffusion is movements of molecules from area of higher concentration to lower concentration. Increased thickness of membranes impedes diffusion. Surface area also can be altered with disease. Oxygen is transported by hemoglobin, molecules combine with oxygen and carbon dioxide. Combination is easily reversible. Carbon dioxide diffuses into RBC and

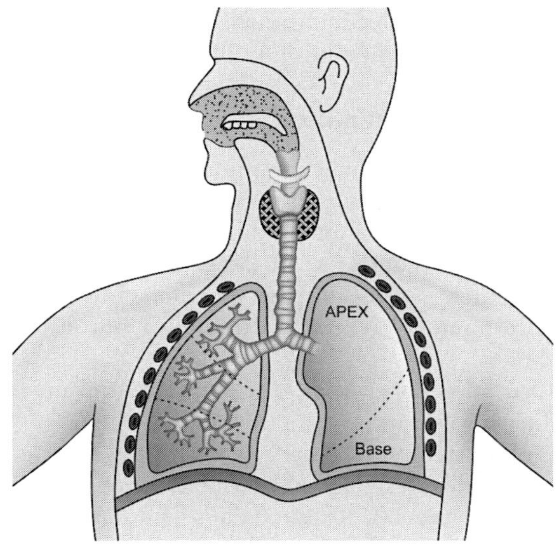

Fig. 10.22: Respiratory system

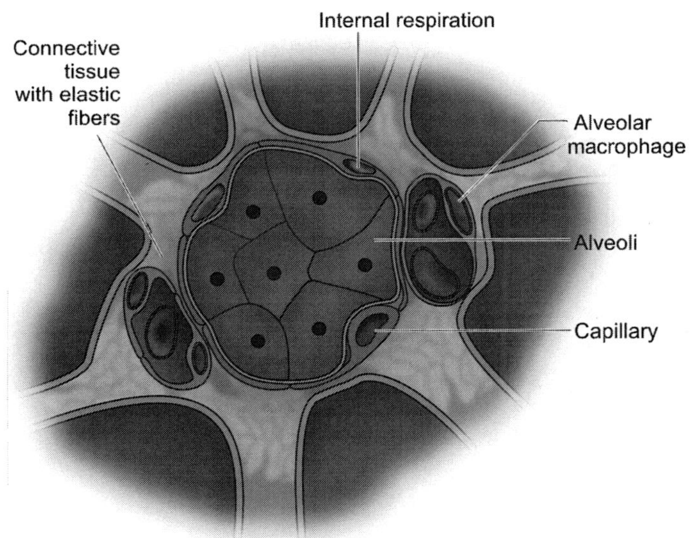

Fig. 10.23: Exchange of gases

rapidly hydrated into carbonic acid. Neural and chemical receptors control and regulate process of respiration (Fig. 10.22).

Factors Affecting Oxygenation

- Physiological factors—conduction disorders of heart, impaired valve function, myocardial hypoxia, cardiomyopathy, respiratory disorders, oxygen carrying capacity of blood, fever, infections, pregnancy, abdominal enlargement due to disease and obesity. Anemia causing decreased oxygen carrying capacity, carbon monoxide poisoning, decreased inspired oxygen concentration, hypovolemia, increased metabolic rate
- Musculoskeletal abnormalities, diseases of central nervous system, spinal column
- Trauma—rib fracture, abdominal incision
- Neuromuscular diseases—myasthenia, polio, multiple sclerosis
- Central nervous system (CNS) alterations—unconsciousness, seizures, poisoning, raised intracranial pressure
- Chronic diseases like bronchial asthma, bronchiectasis, chronic obstructive pulmonary disease (COPD)
- Cardiac dysfunctions—sinus tachycardia, bradycardia, dysrhythmia,
- Altered cardiac output—left ventricular failure, right heart failure (RHF), myocardial infarction (MI), angina
- Hyper- and hypoventilation, hypoxia.

Assessment for Oxygenation

- Review of drugs, food, allergies
- Review of laboratory data on respiratory and ventilatory parameters
- Pain, fatigue, smoking, dyspnea, orthopnea, cough, wheezing
- Increased pCO_2, decreased vital capacity
- Hypoxia, neck vein distension, hydration
- Cyanosis of fingertips, nail beds
- Chest retraction and asymmetry
- Lung sounds, airway patency.

Maintenance of Patent Airway

Airway is patent when trachea, bronchi and large airways are free from obstruction. It requires adequate hydration to prevent thick tenacious mucus secretions. Proper coughing technique removes secretions and keep the airway open. Suctioning, chest physiotherapy, nebulizer therapy helps to maintain clear airway.

Mobilizing pulmonary secretions promote lung expansion and gas exchange. Humidification, proper temperature of water vapor keeps airway moist. Nebulization is process of adding moisture to inspired air.

Oxygen Administration

Oxygen is administered to prevent or relieve hypoxia. Hypoxia is condition of low concentration of oxygen in the tissues. Impaired tissue oxygenation can be improved with controlled oxygen administration. It should be used only when necessary and treated like a drug because it is expensive and has dangerous side effects. Continuous monitoring is mandatory. Oxygen is highly combustible gas, can cause a fire from open flame or electric instrument. Smoking is prohibited when oxygen is in use. Determine all electric instruments are functioning and grounded.

Oxygen is supplied by oxygen tank or pipe line. Cylinder or tank is always to be placed upright. Regulators are used to control flow. Two types of flow meters are seen (Fig. 10.24).

1. Upright flow meter with flow adjustment valve at the top.
2. Cylinder indicator with flow adjustment handle.

Equipment

A tray containing wolf's bottle in a large bowl, connecting rubber tubes, nasal catheter or oxygen mask (Figs 10.25 and 10.26), water in bowl, swab sticks, boric lotion and sticking plaster.

Procedure

- Collect articles and adjust on the locker of patient. Connect tubes to two glass tubes in wolf bottle. Tube connected to the long arm is attached to the cylinder (Fig. 10.24) and tube connected to short arm, nasal catheter is attached which goes to patient's nostril
- Explain the procedure to patient
- Clean the nostrils with boric lotion
- Start the oxygen flow, dip the catheter in water, adjust the flow 3–4 liters if flow meter is not available count the bubbles 40 per minute
- Insert the nasal catheter into nostril
- Ask the patient how he is feeling
- Fix the catheter on patient's forehead or cheek.

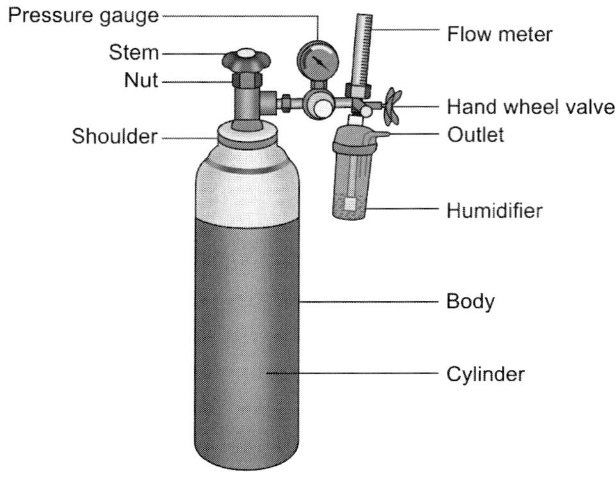

Fig. 10.24: Oxygen apparatus

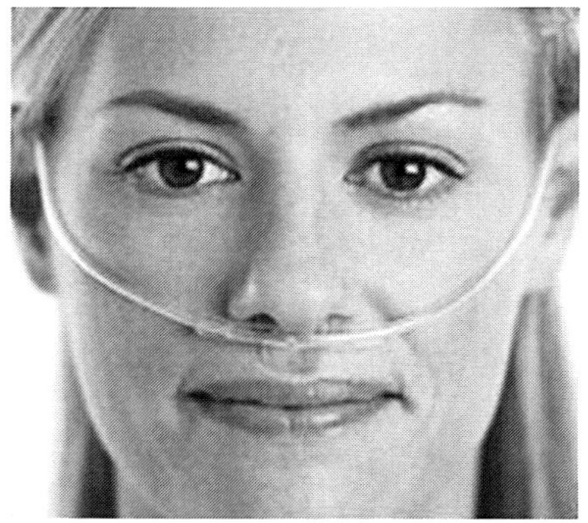

Fig. 10.25: Oxygen by nasal catheter

SUCTION

Suctioning is technique used to clear airway.

Types

- Oropharyngeal
- Nasopharyngeal

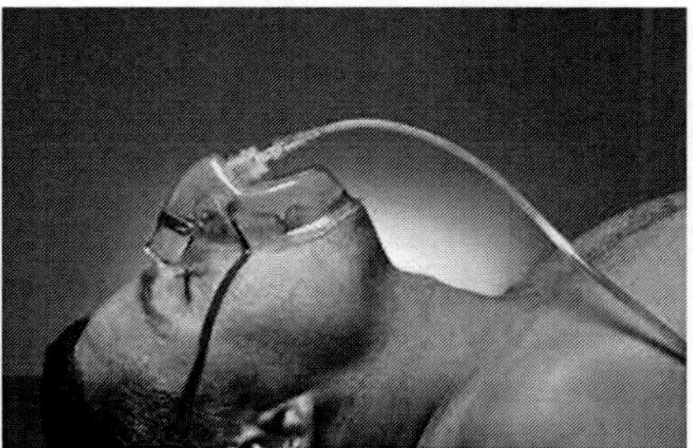

Fig. 10.26: Oxygen by mask

- Orotracheal
- Nasotracheal.

Oropharynx and trachea are considered sterile. Sterile technique is used. Mouth is considered clean.

Suction should be performed after tracheal and oropharyngeal suction. Use of rounded catheter with number of side holes at the distal end of the catheter is made. It should be done according to need. Too frequent suctioning can produce hypoxemia, hypotension, arrhythmias and trauma to mucous membrane.

Insert catheter during inhalation. Never apply suction when inserting catheter. Apply intermittent suction, 10–15 seconds. Replace oxygen device, if present.

Tracheal suctioning: It is done through endotracheal tube or tracheostomy tube. Intermittent suction is applied and catheter is withdrawn. Pressure should be 120–180 mm of Hg. Wear sterile mask and gloves.

Use sterile catheter. Two methods are used. Open and close. Clients on mechanical ventilation require continuous oxygen when suctioning is done.

Equipment

Suction catheter, airway if needed, gloves, towel, portable suction, machine or wall suction, mask, sterile saline 30 mL, connecting tube, Y adapter, water soluble lubricant, basin sterile with 100 mL water or saline.

Procedure

Determine factors like fluid status, lack of humidity, infection, anatomy. Assess client's understanding. Obtain physician's order, if indicated. Explain the procedure to client. Encourage coughing.

Place the patient in comfortable position. Sitting upright or Fowler's position.

Place pulse oximeter on client's finger. Take a reading. Place towel across the chest and wash hands.

Open the suction kit or catheter with aseptic technique. Keep basin with saline on side. Connect tubing to suction. Check suction by sucking water. Set regulator to appropriate pressure. Wall suction, 80–120 mm of Hg. Portable, 7–15 mm of Hg.

Pick up suction catheter, and secure catheter to tubing without touching the catheter to unsterile field.

Check by sucking small amount of saline. Apply 2–3 inches lubricant. If oxygen is given, remove and gently insert the catheter into nares. Do intermittent suction for 10–15 seconds by placing and releasing thumb over catheter vent. Withdraw catheter by rotating it back forth between thumb and forefinger. For nasotracheal suction, insert catheter 16–20 cm for adults.

Deep breathing exercise: A patient is assessed for his normal breathing pattern. To carry out deep breathing exercises person is asked to take 4–5 deep breaths (diaphragmatic). Following last inspiration the person is asked to cough forcefully to expel any secretions. To teach diaphragmatic deep breathing, patient is asked to take deep inspiration and helped by pushing up abdomen against the hand kept.

Deep breathing exercises are helpful in normal life, respiratory difficulty and postoperatively to prevent lung complications.

Chest physiotherapy: It is to mobilize pulmonary secretions in cases of sputum more than 30 mL per day and atelectasis in X-ray. It consists of postural drainage, chest percussions and vibration, productive coughing and suctioning.

Chest percussion: Striking chest wall over the areas being drained. Hand is cupped. Percussion on chest wall sends waves through chest. It changes consistency and location of sputum. It is done over a single layer of clothing excluding buttons, zippers, snaps. Percuss lung area and not scapula. It is contraindicated in bleeding disorders, osteoporosis, fracture ribs. Vibration—fine shaking pressure is applied to chest wall only during expiration. It is used in cystic fibrosis. Contraindicated in children and infants.

Postural Drainage

Use of positioning techniques that drain secretions from specific segment of lung (Figs 10.27A to D).

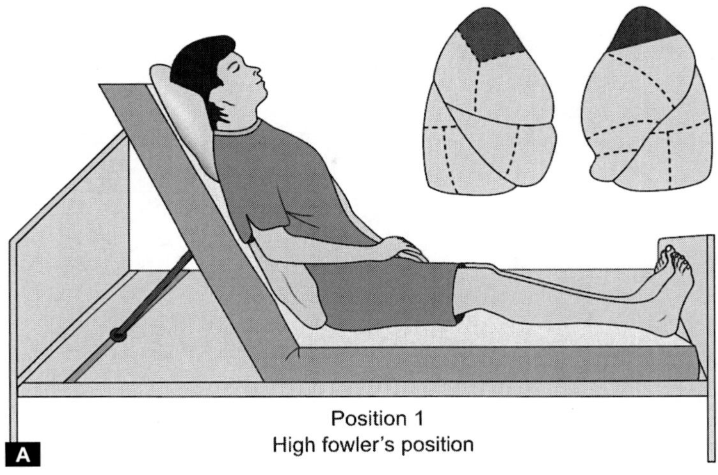

Position 1
High fowler's position

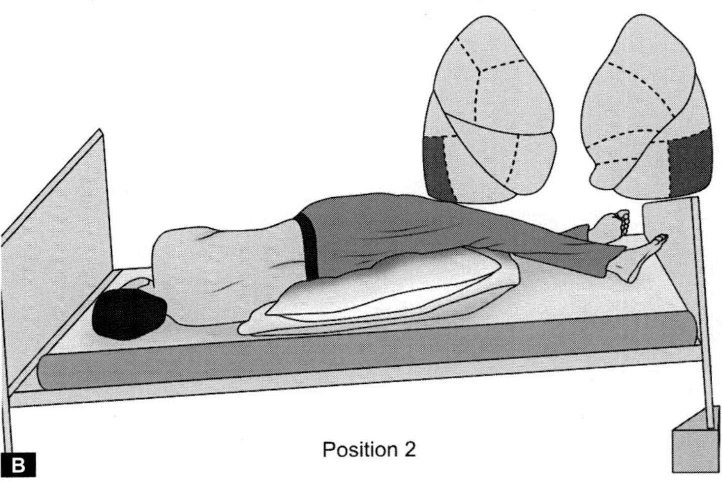

Position 2

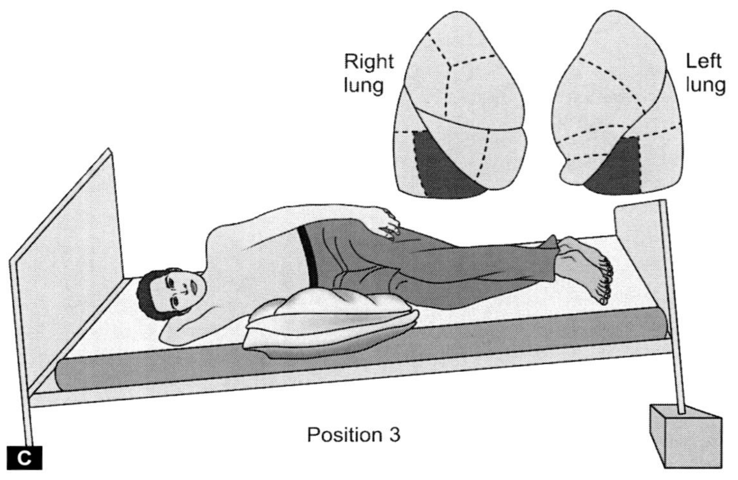

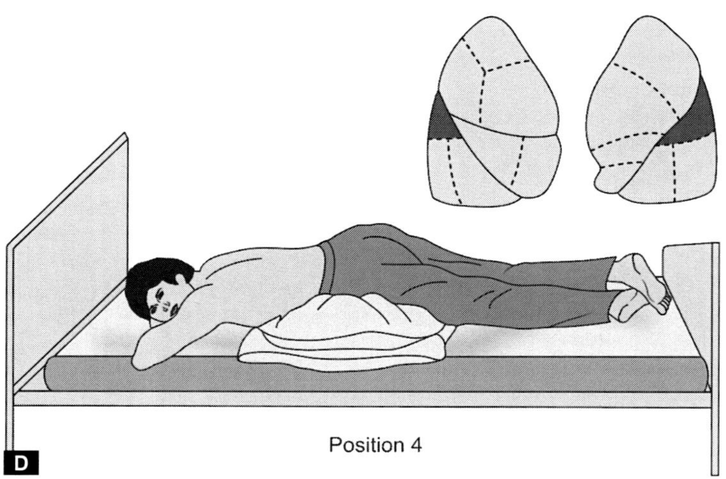

Figs 10.27A to D: Postural drainage

Positions in Postural Drainage

- High Fowler's position
- Supine with head elevated
- Side lying with right side elevated
- Side lying with left side elevated
- ¾ Supine position with dependent lung in Trendelenburg position
- Prone with thorax and abdomen elevated
- Supine in Trendelenburg position
- Right side lying in Trendelenburg position.

Care of Chest Drainage

Chest tube: It is a catheter inserted through the thorax to remove fluid and air.

- Disposable waterless system
- Reusable three glass bottle system
- Mobile chest drain.

Tubes are used after chest surgery, chest trauma, empyema, pneumothorax, hemothorax.

To promote lung expansion: In simple closed drainage system, chamber collects and gives water seal. Fluid goes upon inspiration and comes in chamber on expiration. Two chamber system is also used. Air flows into water sealed chamber and liquid flows in collection chamber. Three chamber system is used when volume of air or fluid needs to be evacuated. Suction is applied 15–20 cm of water.

Precautions

- Always keep below the level of client's chest
- No clamping when client is walking or being transferred
- If tubing disconnects, ask patient to exhale and cough
- Clean and reconnect immediately
- If collecting bag is broken keep the tube end in water.

Care

- Wash hands and assess for chest pain, breath sounds, respiratory distress, vital signs
- Observe site surrounding tube insertion and dressing and tube for kinks, clots, dependent loops, position of drainage system

- Maintain tube connection between chest drainage and tubes intact and taped
- Water sealed vent must be without occlusion and when suction is used suction control chamber vent must be patent
- Adjust tubing to hang straight from top of mattress to drainage chamber
- Mention the time of drainage begun on bottle by adhesive tape
- Milking of tube or stripping is done, if needed and allowed
- To check in water seal system there is bubbling on inspiration and expiration
- Note color and amount of drainage, vital signs, skin color
- Auscultate lungs and observe for symmetry
- Check for leak, proper draining
- Wash hands.

PULSE OXIMETRY

It is noninvasive method of monitoring oxygen saturation of hemoglobin (SpO_2 or SaO_2). It is used when oxygen saturation monitoring is needed in home, clinic, ambulatory setting and hospital. A probe or sensor is attached to fingertip, forehead, earlobe and bridge of nose. Light signals generated are monitored. Normal values are 95–100%. Value less than 85% indicates that tissues are not receiving enough oxygen. Values are unreliable in cases of shock, cardiac arrest, vasoconstriction, severe anemia or high carbon dioxide level.

Cardiopulmonary resuscitation (CPR): It is a basic emergency procedure of artificial respiration and manual external cardiac massage. ABC of CPR is establish airway, initiate breathing, and maintain circulation. Loosen clothes, proper head position, lift jaw, remove obstruction in air passage. Give artificial respiration—mouth-to-mouth, Ambu bag. Chest compression and give cardiac massage.

FLUID ELECTROLYTE AND ACID-BASE BALANCE

Review of Physiological Regulation of Body Fluids, Electrolytes and Acid-base Balance

Homeostasis: It is a process by which body fluid balance is maintained. Regulation is by fluid intake, hormonal control and fluid output.

Fluid intake: Hypothalamus contains thirst control center. It senses the osmolality through osmoreceptors and when it is increased thirst is felt.

Intake of salt, hypertonic fluids, less fluid intake by mouth can increase osmolality and when excess fluid is lost due to vomiting, diarrhea, hemorrhage results in hypovolemia.
Usually 2200–2700 mL, fluid is taken daily by an adult.

Hormonal Control

Antidiuretic hormone of posterior pituitary gland prevents diuresis and reabsorption is increased which again enters systemic circulation. Aldosteron a hormone by adrenal cortex acts on distal tubules increases reabsorption of sodium and excretion of potassium. Sodium retains water. Renin acts to produce angiotensin I which causes vasoconstriction. Angiotensin II causes selective vasoconstriction later on, and increases blood flow to kidneys and stimulates aldosteron.

Fluid Output

Kidneys, skin, lungs and gastrointestinal tract are organs which excrete fluids. Kidneys filter plasma 120 mL/minute, 180 L/day and produce 1200–1500 mL of urine. Skin excretes 500–600 mL of fluid. Lungs lose 400 mL fluid from expiration. 100–200 mL water is lost from gastrointestinal tract (GI). 3000–6000 mL fluid is secreted and reabsorbed by gastrointestinal tract.
Regulation of electrolytes—Major cations within body fluids are Na^+, K^+, Ca^{++}, Mg^{++}. When one cation leaves the cell, other enters. Na^+ is required for osmolality, nerve impulse transmission and regulation of acid-base balance. It is regulated by dietary intake and aldosteron secretion.
K^+: It is intracellular cation 98% and 2% in extracellular fluid (ECF). It regulates metabolic processes. It is required for glycogen deposit, conduction of nerve impulse, smooth muscles contractions, normal cardiac rhythm. Normal concentration in blood is 3.5–5 mEq/L. It is regulated by dietary intake and excreted by kidney.
Ca^{++}: It is stored in bones, plasma, body cells. Bones—99% ECF—1%, normal serum.

Ionized calcium is 4–5 mEq/L. Its function is formation of bones and teeth, clotting of blood, hormone secretion, cell membrane integrity, cardiac conduction, nerve impulse and muscle contraction.
Mg^{++}: It is essential for enzyme activities, neurochemical activities, cardiac and skeletal muscles excitability. Plasma contains 1.5–2.5 mEq/L. Dietary intake, parathyroid hormone, kidneys regulate Mg^{++} balance.

Major anions in body fluids are Cl^-, HCO_3^-, PO3/4—Chloride, bicarbonate, phosphate.

Extracellular fluid contains 95–108 mEq/L chloride (serum) and is excreted by kidneys. Bicarbonate is found in extracellular fluid (ECF) and intracellular fluid (ICF). It is necessary for acid-base balance.

Kidney regulates bicarbonates. Phosphate helps in acid-base balance.

Acid-base Balance

It is balance between various acids produced in body in metabolic process and excretion of the same. H^+ ion concentration if more, it is acidic and if HCO_3 ion concentration is more, it is base. The balance is always maintained by three buffer systems of the body, kidneys, lungs and hemoglobin.

Factors Affecting Fluid Electrolyte and Acid-base Balance

Factors affecting osmolality

- Free water loss
- Diabetes insipidus
- Sodium overload
- Hyperglycemia
- Uremia
- Fluid volume deficit
- Acidosis
- Renal failure
- Diuretics
- Adrenal insufficiency
- Fluid volume excess
- Syndrome of inappropriate antidiuretic hormone (SIADH).

Alterations in Fluids Electrolyte and Acid-base Balance

- Fluid volume deficit (FVD)
- Fluid volume excess
- Acidosis—Metabolic and respiratory
- Alkalosis
- Hypokalemia
- Hyperkalemia
- Hyponatremia
- Hypernatremia.

Nursing Interventions

Assessment

Fluid volume deficit (FVD): Monitor and measure fluid intake and output 8 hourly and sometimes hourly when required.

Fluid loss may be from excessive urination, vomiting, diarrhea, excessive perspiration (Diaphoresis). FVD is when urine output is less than 30 mL/hour, daily body weight is recorded. 0. 5 kg wt loss = 500 mL fluid loss.

Monitor vital signs: Weak rapid pulse, postural hypotension, decrease in body temperature. Monitor skin turgor and tongue. Skin flattens very slowly or may remain elevated when pinched. Pinch the skin over sternum, inner thigh or forehead. Look for additional long furrows on tongue and size is small. Dry mouth and lips. Measure specific gravity of urine. Cold extremities due to decreased peripheral perfusion. Low central venous pressure (CVP). Prevent FVD by identifying risk and take measures to minimize fluid loss. Oral fluids, medication ordered.

Fluid volume excess: Isotonic expansion of ECF by retention of water and sodium.

Edema, distended neck veins, crackles, tachycardia, hypertension, increased CVP, increased weight, increased urine output, shortness of breath and wheezing.

Measuring fluid intake and output—measure intake and output for patients after surgery, patients with unstable conditions, patients on fluid restriction, fever, on diuretics and IV therapy, having blood transfusion, and renal disease.

Intake: All liquids taken by mouth—water, juice, soup, ice cream, gelatin, fluids, milk, liquids given through nasogastric tube, IV fluids, blood or its components.

Output: Urine, diarrhea, vomit, gastric suction, drainage from wounds and tubes. Ask the patient to save urine in graduated container. For aspiration, catheter in bladder, record output at the end of each shift or hourly.

Correcting Fluid Electrolyte Balance

Assessment: Monitor arterial blood gas (ABG) levels, vital signs, intake and output, weight and oxygen saturation levels.

Mucous membrane, auscultate breath sounds, palpate skin turgor. Ask if client is thirsty or weak. Observe for abnormal loss of fluid. Assess client's tolerance to changing from lying to sitting position.

Nursing diagnosis: Fluid volume deficit.

Outcome: The client will demonstrate fluid balance by moist mucous membranes, balanced intake output measurements, stable daily weight. Client will be free of complications associated with the IV device, throughout the duration of IV therapy.

Replacement of fluids: Oral—juice, soup, milk, water, coconut water, congee, dal water.

Whey, buttermilk, other drinks, ice cream, ice, tea, coffee, cold drinks, albumin water, oral rehydration solution.

Parenteral: Dextrose 5%, normal saline, ringer lactate.

Venipuncture: Insertion of a needle into vein for the introduction of drug or fluid or for the withdrawal of blood (Figs 10.28 and 10.29).

Purpose

- To collect blood for laboratory tests
- To start IV line for intravenous infusion of fluids
- To inject drugs.

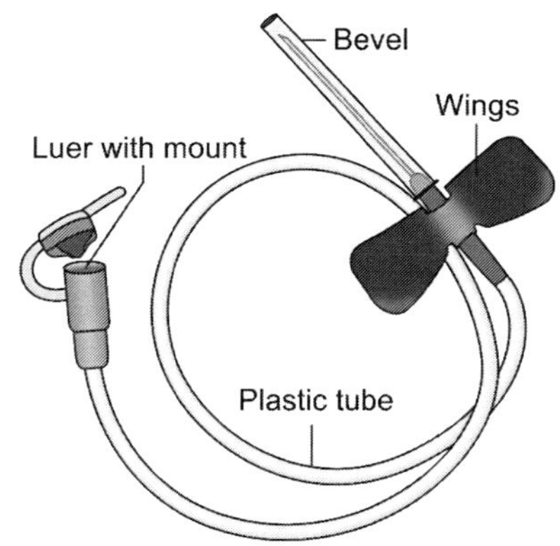

Fig. 10.28: Scalp vein needle

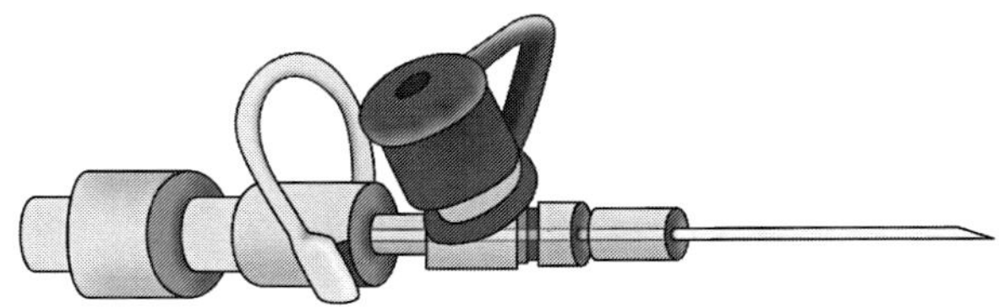

Fig. 10.29: Venipuncture cannula

Equipment: Sterile disposable syringe and needle, betadine or spirit swab, specimen bottles, drugs to be injected, tourniquet, gloves, mackintosh, splint, if needed.

Procedure: Place mackintosh and small napkin under patient's elbow. Wash hands with soap and water. Wear gloves. Explain the procedure to client. Palpate and select vein. Common sites are cephalic, basilica and median cubital veins. Use most distal site, avoid painful areas, avoid fragile veins in old people. Apply tourniquet. Clean insertion site with swab in firm circular motion. Allow it to dry. Perform venipuncture by placing thumb over vein beneath the insertion site and stretching skin against direction of insertion. Warn client of sharp stick. Puncture skin and vein and collect blood samples. Release tourniquet. Inject drug, if ordered. Start IV line if not seal or press the site after removing needle. Wash hands. Remove gloves. Wash hands. Make client comfortable.

Intravenous infusion: It is an introduction of fluid into vein.

Equipment: Infusion set depending on type of infusion, rate of administration. Extension tubing if needed, betadine or spirit swab, gloves, tourniquet or rubber tubing, arm board if needed, towel, tape, IV stand, special gown with snaps at shoulder if available, sterile gauze piece, precut tape.

For heparin or normal saline, lock-injection cap, short piece of IV tubing, 1–3 mL of normal saline or heparin flush 10–100 μ/mL, syringe and 25 No. needle.

Procedure

- Check physician's order for amount and type of fluid
- Observe signs of imbalance, previous IV therapy, arm used and whether he is going to receive blood transfusion later on
- Assess laboratory data, history of allergies
- Assess for risk factors—age, child or old age, heart or renal failure, low platelet count
- Explain the purpose and procedure to patient and relative
- Assist and give sitting or supine position
- Wash hands
- Organize equipment
- Wear gown, if available
- Open sterile package with aseptic technique
- Check IV solution using 5 rights
- Make sure additives like potassium, vitamins are added. Check clarity, expiry date before adding
- Insert IV tube in port

- Open infusion set. Place roller clamp, 2–5 cm below chamber to off position
  - Hang at 36 inches
  - Start flow, expel air, regulate the flow, connect to needle at venipuncture.

Regulating Intravenous Flow Rate

- Check the solution for correctness. Observe for patency of IV line
- Open drip regulator and observe rapid flow and close the drip to prescribed rate
- Compress cannulated vein slightly proximal to end of tube and observe drip chamber
- Ask the client about his understanding of position of arm affecting IV flow
- Ask if he has burning sensation or pain
- Calculate, know calibrations in drops per milliliter of infusion set. microdrip—60 drops per mL and macrodrip—15 drops per milliliter or 10 drops per milliliter
- Select one of the formulas.
  - $\text{mL/hr} = \dfrac{\text{Total infusion}}{\text{Hours of infusion}}$
  - mL/hr/60 minutes = mL/mn ileus

  Drop factor × mL/mn = drops/mn
  3000 mL/24 hours =125 mL/hr/60=2.1 mL/mn
  125 mL/hr × 20 drops/mL/60 = 125 × 20 = 2500/60 =
  41 drops/mn = 2 mL/mn
- Count drops for minute
- Increase or decrease rate.

Changing Intravenous Solution and Tubing

- Venus dressing—Keep the system sterile. Never disconnect tubing
- Insert IV tube in port. Do not expose port to air
- Change before solution runs out, prepare when 50 mL solution remains
- Explain the procedure and purpose to client
- Wash hands, prepare new solution
- Remove protective cover from IV tubing port, move roller clamp to stop flow
- Remove old container from stand and quickly

remove spike from old solution bag and without touching tip insert spike into new bag or bottle

- Hang new bag or bottle. Check for air in tubing
  If air present, remove by closing roller clamp. For large amount of air insert syringe into port below the air and aspirate. Swab port with 70% alcohol and allow it to dry before inserting needle
- Ensure drip chamber is only half or one-third full
- If too full, pinch off tubing below drip chamber and invert container and squeeze drip chamber. Hang the bottle and release the clamp and regulate the flow.

BLOOD REPLACEMENT OR TRANSFUSION

It is intravenous administration of whole blood or its components like plasma, packed cells or platelets.

Purpose

- To increase volume of circulating blood
- To increase red blood cells
- To provide selected cellular component.

Indications: Surgery, trauma, hemorrhage, severe anemia, replacement of clotting factor, albumin, platelets.

Grouping and cross matching: Blood group is identified and blood to be transfused is crossmatched with client's blood. Rh factor is also determined. Blood is tested for HIV and HBV.

Autologous transfusion is collection of client's own blood. Transfusing blood is nursing procedure.

If IV line is present, assess venipuncture (Fig. 10.29) site for infection or infiltration. See gauge of IV catheter 18–19 is preferred. See for patency and functioning. Fill the tube with normal saline to prevent hemolysis. If not, start IV line. Ask for previous transfusion and reaction, if any.

Explain the procedure. Instruct to report if any chills, dizziness, fever. Obtain baseline vital signs.

Ensure right client, compatibility of blood. Check label on blood product, blood group and complete name. Start slowly, monitor side effects, stay for 15 minutes. Observe vital signs periodically. When rapid transfusions are needed give through central venous catheter. If transfusion reaction is anticipated, monitor vital signs more frequently.

Transfusion Reactions

It is systemic reaction of the body to incompatible blood.
Causes: Red cell incompatibility, allergy to blood components transfused, allergy to preservative and infected blood.
Risks: Disease like AIDS, hepatitis, malaria, may be transmitted, if serological testing is not done.

Circulatory overload in older adults and clients with cardiopulmonary disease. These reactions are life-threatening. If reaction is suspected, stop the transfusion, call doctor, monitor vital signs, keep ready drugs like antihistaminic, vasopressors, steroids. Prepare for CPR, collect urine specimen and send it to laboratory. Keep blood, tubings, labels transfusion record and send to laboratory.

RESTRICTION OF FLUIDS

Client's with fluid volume excess, require restricted fluids. Allow half of the total allotted oral fluid from 7 am to 3 pm.

Give frequent oral care. Explain the client the reason to restrict the fluids. Keep daily intake output and weight chart. Weight should be taken daily at same time and on the same weighing scale after client voids.

PSYCHOLOGICAL NEEDS—ASSESSMENT

- Love and belonging
- Safety and security
- Self-esteem
- Resources identification
- Family support
- Hope, trust, industry, integrity, bonding
- Values, right attitude, beliefs about life
- Sources of guidance
- Stressors, coping, loss
- Emotional control, maturity, stability.

Assessment can be done through observation, interview of patient and relatives. Behaviors like withdrawal, attention seeking, exacerbating, anger, crying, refusing, avoiding, temper, tantrums, etc. Nonverbal communications through facial expressions, gestures indicating fear, anxiety, irritability, anger, tension, etc. Situational low self-esteem, disturbed sleep pattern, caregiver role strain, fear, chronic pain, powerlessness can be assessed.

THERAPEUTIC ENVIRONMENT

Recreation and Diversional Therapy

Therapeutic environment provides cleanliness, comfort, equipments for various treatments, recreation and diversional activities.

- Music—Soft music spreading positive feelings, inspiration and optimism helps to recover from disease
- Play—Play therapy especially for children individually or in group. Play material like wooden blocks, colorful toys of rubber and fur (animals, doll)
- Television and Newspapers
- Reading material—religious, cultural, fictions, books, magazines
- Cassettes and CD
- Storytelling, puppet show, craft work, paper work, drawing, painting
- Sand and water, mud playing.

NURSING INTERVENTIONS FOR PSYCHOLOGICAL NEEDS

- Developing trust
- Professional behavior
- Emotional support
- Creating hope
- Developing value of life
- Motivating and encouraging
- Providing safe environment
- Assistance in ADL
- Meeting specific needs which create stress, e.g. colostomy care, loss of body part
- Promoting self-dependences
- Promoting self-image and self-esteem
- Provide communication devices.

STRESS AND ADAPTATION

Stress is universal part of human experience. It is necessary for survival. It provides stimulation and motivation. It causes discomfort and retreat. Fight or flight response to stress is arousal of sympathetic nervous system.

This reaction prepares a person for action by increasing heart rate, diverting blood to brain and muscles, increasing blood pressure, respiratory rate and blood sugar levels.

General Adaptation Syndrome

It is immediate physiological response of the body to stress and involves mainly autonomic and endocrine systems of body. It is initiated by pituitary. Hypothalamus secretes endorphins which are hormones that act on mind like sedation and reducing pain. During alarm reaction, hormone level rises increasing blood volume, glucose level, adrenaline oxygen intake, mental alertness, blood flow to brain and muscles. Pupils dilate. Resistance Stage—Body stabilizes and responds. Increased rates come to normal. Body repairs the damage. If still stress remains then, exhaustion stage—body can no longer resist. Energy level is diminished. Physiological regulation diminishes and if stress still continues death may occur.

Types of Stress

Distress: Damaging stress
Eustress: Protecting stress—work stress, family stress, acute or chronic stress, daily hassles, trauma
Crisis are some of the examples of stress.

CHAPTER

11

Infection Control in Clinical Setting

AIM

Students are able to practice aseptic technique and use measures to control infection in clinical setting.

OBJECTIVES

- Students are able to explain difference between medical and surgical asepsis
- Perform proper hand hygiene
- Explain nature, chain of infection and defense against infection
- Explain about nosocomical infections and precautions to prevent
- Explain about biomedical waste and its management.

NATURE OF INFECTION

An infection is the entry and multiplication of an infectious agent in the tissues of the host. If pathogen fails to cause injury to tissues, it is colonizing the tissue without causing harm.

If the disease can be transmitted directly from one person to another it is communicable. Patients with communicable disease and infectious that are easily transmissible to others require special precautions.

Systemic infections are those that affect the whole body and require measures to prevent complications of fever. Localized infections require removal of infectious organisms, e.g. application of dry and wet dressing, insertion of drainage tube.

Use medical and surgical aseptic techniques and ensure correct handling of infected drainage or body fluids.

Chain in Infection Transmission

Infectious Agents

Bacteria, viruses, fungi, protozoa microorganisms on skin are called resident or transient flora. They are not easily removed by plain hand washing. Antimicrobial soaps are required to remove bacteria from deeper layer of the skin. Transient microorganism attach to the skin when person touches person or object, to enter and survive in the host, susceptibility of the host.

Reservoir

Place where pathogen can survive but may or may not multiply, e.g. Human body.

Carriers

Persons or animals that show no illness but bear pathogen which can be transferred to others.

Portal of Exit

Skin, respiratory tract, urinary tract, GI tract, reproductive tract and blood.

Mode of Transmission

- **Contact**
  - **Direct:** Person to person, physical contact, fecal-oral
  - **Indirect:** Through contaminated objects, needles, dressings
  - **Droplet:** Coughing, sneezing, talking
- **Air:** Droplets suspended in air after coughing, sneezing carried on dust particles
- **Vehicles:** Contaminated articles, water, drugs, solutions blood, food
- **Vector:** Flies, parasites.
  Vector and host—mosquito, louse, flea, tick.

Portal of entry: Exit routes can be used for entry. Prick injury, abrasion, and ingestion, through inhalation, ascending urinary infection from urinary catheter, wound, ulcer, and burns.

Defense against Infection

Natural

Respiratory system is lined with ciliated epithelium. Rhythmic movements of these prevent entry of microorganisms, these move flow of mucus and trap organisms and throw into pharynx for removal.

Hydrochloric acid in the stomach protects from ingested bacteria. Sense of small and odor, taste prevents eating infected material.

Body's cellular response to injury or infection is inflammation. It is protective vascular reaction that delivers fluid, blood products and nutrients to interstitial tissues in an area of injury. Process neutralizes and eliminates pathogen.

Intact, multilayered skin provides barrier to microorganisms. Shedding of outer layer and sebum removes organisms adherent. Saliva washes away particles containing microbes. Tearing and blinking reduces entry of microbes. Flushing action of urine flow washes away microbes. Intact multilayered mucous membrane prevents entry of organisms.

Acidic pH in vagina prevents entry of organisms and their growth.

Hospital Acquired Infection

(Nosocomial infection)

Nosocomial infections result from healthcare systems and workers.

Types

Iatrogenic: It results from diagnostic or therapeutic procedures.

Exogenous: Microorganisms external to the individual.

Endogenous: Clients bacterial flora can become source of infection.

Sources of Infection

- Contaminated hands
- Contaminated equipment
- Health personnel with infections
- Client with infectious diseases.

Preventing Nosocomial Infections

- Health checkup and treatment of infection in health workers
- Sterilization and asepsis
- Hand hygiene and standard precautions

- Isolation of infectious clients
- Barrier nursing
- Protective attire
- Disinfection and proper disposal of waste
- Infection control committee
- Sending swabs to laboratory and fumigation.

BASIC CONCEPTS IN MEDICAL AND SURGICAL ASEPSIS

Concepts

Preventing cross infection and nosocomical infections requires practice of medical and surgical asepsis, on the basis of principles of microbiology, sterilization, aseptic technique, disinfection and standard precautions.

Terminology

- **Asepsis:** Freedom from pathogenic organisms
- **Antiseptics:** Any substance that prevents growth of bacteria
- **Disinfection:** Killing of pathogenic organisms with chemical substances such as glutaraldehyde, sodium hypochlorite or phenol
- **Disinfectants:** Any agent that destroys infection producing organisms or pathogenic organisms
- **Contamination:** Act of soiling by contact
- **Cross infection:** Contagion—the communication of disease from one person to another by direct contact
- **Nosocomial infection:** Infection acquired in hospital, at least 72 hours after admission. Also called as hospital acquired infection.

  Contact transmitted infection is the most important and frequent mode of transmission of nosocomial infections and may be either direct or indirect

  Direct: Body surface to body surface contact, e.g. patient being the source of infection and other susceptible host.

  Indirect: Indirect contact transmitted infections involve contact of susceptible host with contaminated intermediate object usually inanimate, e.g. Instruments, needles, dressings, gloves that are not changed between patients. Unwashed contaminated hands may also be source of nosocomial infection
- **Sterile:** Free of organisms.

Handling Sterile Articles

- Sterile articles are always kept above waistline and in front and not at the back, when standing as they are considered contaminated, if below waistline and at the back
- Never touch sterile articles with bare hands as hands are considered as clean and not sterile
- Use sterile forceps or cheatle forceps for handling. Do not drop fluid from these forceps, always hold forceps pointing down because if you hold pointing up, the fluid will run down along the forceps towards hand and again while holding, pointing downwards fluid will come down from hand to the tip contaminating it
- Never let the water dribble from the end to handle, side and back to the hand
- Keep sterile drum closed and apertures closed
- Never assume that object is sterile
- Avoid sweeping, dusting when sterile articles are opened
- Keep unsterile objects away from sterile field
- Keep sterile field dry
- Invert cover when you want to place it down
- When opening sterile pack, edges should be directed away as edges are considered unsterile
- Do not speak, sneeze or cough over sterile pack
- Open farthest flap first when opening sterile pack
- Do not touch sterile articles with unsterile forceps or contaminated articles
- Pour only required amount of solution so that it is not wasted (for dressing)
- Put a sterile towel to prepare sterile field
- Once the articles are sterilized they are sterile for 72 hours. If not used, are to be sent for sterilization again.

BARRIER METHODS OF PATIENT CARE

Care of Hands

- If open wounds are present on hands or arms of the health worker, they should be properly covered with waterproof dressing
- While handling/processing blood or body fluids, the health worker should always wear gloves

- At the end of the procedure, the gloved hands should be dipped in 1% hypochlorite solution and then washed thoroughly with soap and water
- Then the gloves should be removed taking care that the exterior surface of the gloves does not come in contact with the hands or body
- The gloves should be put in 1% hypochlorite solution
- Hands and arms as well as other parts of the body exposed to infected material should be washed with soap and water after removal of gloves.

ISOLATION TECHNIQUE—BARRIER NURSING

It is to confine the microorganisms within given and recognized area. It prevents cross infection. It is used for infectious patients to prevent pathogenic organisms getting transferred to other patient. Separate hospitals, wards are available for infectious patients for isolation. If isolation unit is used for infectious patient separate equipment and articles are used for that particular patient. Body substances such as feces, saliva, mucus and wound drainage always contain potentially infectious organism. Isolation or barrier precautions include the appropriate use of gowns, gloves, mask, and eyewear and other protective devices and clothing. Barrier protection is indicated for use with all the patients because every patient has potential to transmit infection via blood, body fluids.

Airborne, droplet and contact precautions based on diagnosis of the patient.

Regardless of type of isolation, nurse has to take the following precautions:

- Use of hand hygiene before entering and leaving room
- Disposal of contaminated supplies in manner that prevents spread of microorganisms
- Application of knowledge of disease process
- Protection of exposed persons
- When client is isolated in a private room especially children may feel lonely, rejected, and unclean, relatives may be taught regarding disease, specific precautions, environment should be clean
- Isolation room or adjoining room should provide facility for hand washing, bathing, toilet. Soap and antiseptic solutions are made available
- Provide impervious bag for soiled or contaminated linen
- Disposable rigid container should be available in the room to discard needles, syringes and sharp objects
- Stethoscopes, BP apparatus, thermometers used for isolation patients should not be used for others unless they are disinfected

- Gown, gloves, mask, protective eyewear should be available for personnel caring for client
- Gowning prevents soiling clothes during contact with client usually made up of fluid resistant material and to be changed if damaged or heavily contaminated
- Isolation gowns open at the back and ties are at neck and waist to secure and keep closed
- Gown should be long enough to cover all outer garments
- Mask protects from inhaling microorganisms. Full face mask is to be worn when anticipates splashing or spraying of blood or body fluid. Surgical mask protects nurse from inhalation of organisms from respiratory tract of client and transmission of pathogen from nurse's respiratory tract to the client. It also prevents suspended particles in air from inhaling, properly applied mask fits over mouth and nose snugly
- Gloves help to prevent transmission of pathogen by direct and indirect contact. Clean, nonsterile gloves should be worn when touching blood, body fluid, secretions, excretions and contaminated items. Clean gloves should be donned just before touching mucous membrane and nonintact skin. Gloves should be changed between tasks and procedures on the same client after contact with material that may contain high concentration of microorganisms. Gloves should be removed promptly after use, before touching non-contaminated items and environmental surfaces and before caring other patients
- Sequence of wearing protective devices is performing hand hygiene, apply mask and eyewear or goggle, wear gown then wear gloves, pull glove cuffs on gown.

Hand Washing

Hand washing helps to remove microorganisms, dirt, and stains in turn prevents cross infection. Hands should be washed thoroughly before and after nursing procedure, caring another patient, leaving the ward and entering the ward. Hand washing must be carried out after removal of protective clothing, between patient contacts, after contact with blood or body fluids, before invasive procedures and before handling food.

Hand Washing Procedure

Wash hands under running water (Fig. 11.1A). Push wristwatch, long sleeves up, remove ring, and adjust water flow. Avoid splashing. Wet hands with water and apply soap or liquid soap from palm to elbow in a circular movement. Keep hands and wrist-lower at level to elbow, make plenty of lather. Interlace fingers and rub palms and back of hands with circular motion at least 5 times each (Fig. 11.1B). Keep fingertips down. Clean finger nails with nails of other hand, additional soap and orange stick wash. Repeat steps, if hands are heavily soiled. Turn off tap with paper napkin if hand touch is used, if pedal operated, turn off with foot. Dry hands with paper napkin, single use towel or air dryer. (Hands are to be washed till they are clean, usually 3–5 minutes and heavily soiled for 7 minutes).

Hand Antisepsis, Surgical Antisepsis (Scrub)

Use of antimicrobial soap (antiseptic) is encouraged when nurses work in special care units, perform invasive procedures, or care patients who are immune compromised, have damage to their integumentary systems (wounds) or are infected with or colonized with epidemiologically significant organisms, e.g. *Staphylococcus aureus* or vancomycin resistant *enterococcus* (VRE).

Antiseptic solutions containing chlorhexidine, glutaraldehyde, alcohol or iodophor are used. Certain antimicrobial soaps can irritate skin.

Surgical Scrub

All hand jewelery including watch is removed, faucets are regulated with elbow, knee or foot control.

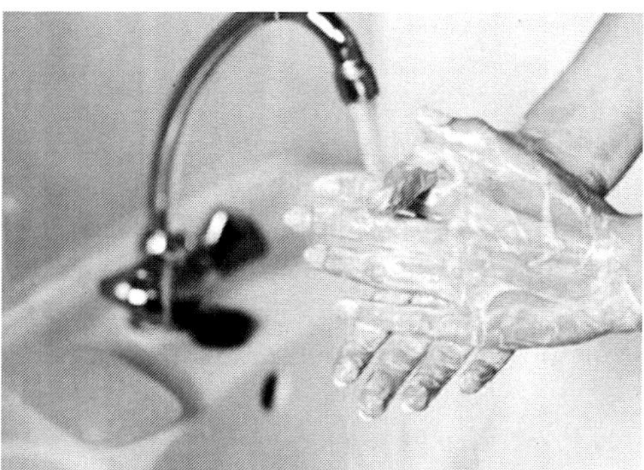

Fig. 11.1A: Hand wash

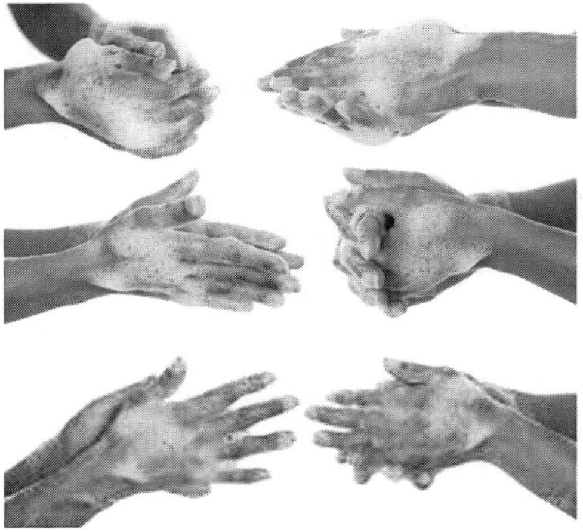

Fig. 11.1B: Hand wash

Liquid antibacterial soap is used. Scrubbing devices may be incorporated with antibacterial soap.

Scrubbing lasts 2–5 minutes, depending on the antibacterial agent and time interval between subsequent scribes. Hands are held higher than the elbows during washing, rinsing and drying. Areas beneath the fingernails are cleaned with an orange stick or nail cleaner. Friction is produced by scrubbing with sponge and hand brush. Hands are dried with sterile towel and sterile gloves are donned immediately after the hands are dried.

Isolation—Source and Protection (Table 11.1)

Table 11.1: Protective isolation of patients and its sources

Source	*Protection*
1. Hands	Hand hygiene, surgical scrub, wearing gloves, decontamination of hands in all clinical situations, alcohol-based waterless antiseptic for routine decontamination
2. Catheters	Closing of drainage bags, aseptic precautions, disinfecting, sterilizing if reused or proper disposal
3. Droplets	Using special mask, ventilated room, standard precautions

Contd...

Contd...

Source	*Protection*
4. Splashing spraying	Full mask, glasses, minimum talking, gown and gloves
5. Specimen collection	Use of disposable gloves, sterile equipment
6. Linen contaminated items	Bagging procedure. Double bagging, if outer surface contamination expected
7. Transport	Clean gown to patient, mask, person transporting should wear gown and mask, extra sheet to cover stretcher or wheel chair
8. Blood, body fluids, dressing swabs	Bagging procedure

Personal

Protecting equipment, types, uses, techniques of wearing and removing gown, mask, protective eyewear and gloves.

Gowning prevents soiling of clothes during contact with clients. It helps to protect from coming in contact with infected material and should be changed immediately, if damaged or heavily soiled and contaminated. They may be disposable or reusable.

Gowns open at back and have ties or snaps to secure at neck and waist. It is long enough to cover outer garments. Long and tight-fitting sleeves and cuffs give more protection.

Carefully removing of gown is needed to minimize contamination of hands, uniform and then discard it. Full-face protection should be worn when splashing or spraying of blood or body fluid or to face is anticipated. Mask should also be worn in airborne and droplet precautions.

- Rational use of gloves.
  - Gloves should be worn while carrying out any invasive procedures as well as while handling infected material
  - Body parts like nose, eyes, skin, hair, of oneself should not be touched with gloved hand by health worker
  - Workplace should not be left wearing gloves
  - Telephone or other items should not be touched with gloved hands.
- Care of gloves—With available resources, we may have to reuse gloves with proper sterilization. Therefore, after any invasive procedure:
  - Gloved hands should be thoroughly washed with hypochlorite solution
  - Then the gloved hands should be rinsed with soap and water
  - The glove should then be removed and kept in 1% hypochlorite solution for 20 minutes for disinfection

- At the end of 20 minutes, they should be washed thoroughly and hanged for drying
- Dried gloves should be tested for presence of holes, etc. by filling each glove with 25 ± 25 mL of water at room temperature and watching for leakage
- Intact, dried gloves should then be sent for 'autoclaving' before reusing them
- Gloves which show holes, cuts, tears, etc. should be discarded
- Gloves should not be disposed without proper disinfections.

Protective Attire

Protective attire should be worn by the health worker whenever splashing or splattering of infected material during any clinical situation is anticipated. Aerosolization or splattering of blood or other infected material issues anticipated during orthopedic surgery or dental surgery wherein highspeed drills are used. To avoid the contamination of skin/ mucous membrane, face mask and protective eyewear should be worn. Splashing of blood is expected during child birth, or cases of massive bleeding due to trauma or crush injuries. In such situation, surgical gown of cotton alone is not adequate, as it would get soaked with blood. Therefore, under such circumstances a waterproof apron should be worn underneath the surgical gown.

Decontamination of Equipment and Unit

When an object comes in contact with infected material, the object gets contaminated. If the object is disposable, it is discarded. Reusable objects must be cleaned thoroughly before reuse and then disinfected or sterilized. Wear mask, eyewear, waterproof gloves, wash under running cold water to remove organic material. After rinsing, wash with soap and water, rinse in warm water. Disinfect in 2% sodium hypochlorite solution. Other disinfectants are alcohols, chlorine, glutaraldehyde and phenols.

Methods of High-Level Disinfections

Simple boiling for 20 minutes to achieve high-level disinfections. The instruments and equipment which cannot be autoclaved or boiled can be disinfected using chemical disinfectant.

The following disinfectants have been known to be in destroying HIV.

- Sodium hypochlorite compounds

- Ethanol 70%
- 2-Propanol (isopropyl alcohol) 70%
- Polyvidone iodine 2.5%
- Formaldehyde 2% (Didex)
- Hydrogen peroxide 6%.

BUSINESS OF CHEMICAL DISINFECTION

Chloride Releasing Compounds

Sodium hypochlorite (Chlorosan) commerical names may differ. Sodium hypochlorite solutions (liquid bleach) are excellent disinfectants which kill bacteria and viruses. They are inexpensive and widely available. However, they are corrosive. They corrode metals and hence cannot be used repeatedly for metallic instruments.

Stock solutions should be recently manufactured and protected from heat and light. Dilutions from stock solutions should be prepared just before use. While disinfections of heavily soiled equipment, blood spills, etc. stronger solutions with a concentration of 1% available chlorine (10 g/L 10,000 ppm) are required.

Dilution of sodium hypochlorite solution.
(Parts of stock sol: Part of water)

Required strength	5% stock	15% stock
0.1 (1 gm/L, 1000 ppm)	Dil: 1:50	Dil: 1:150
1% (10 gm/L, 10000 ppm)	1:5	1:15

Rapid decomposition of tresses solutions may be major problem in countries with a warm climate. Therefore, only freshly solutions should be used.

Chloramines (tosylchloramide sodium, chloramine T) chloramines is more stable than sodium hypochlorite. It should however, be stored and protected from humidity, light band, excessive heat. It is available as powder or tablets. After immersion in sodium hypochlorite all the items/ instruments should be thoroughly washed with water.

Concentrations

The disinfectant power of all chlorine releasing compounds is expressed as available chlorine [0% for solid compound and d% or parts per million (ppm) for solutions] according to the concentration level. Thus,

0.0001% is 1 mg/L = 1 ppm and d% = 10 gm/L = 10,000 ppm. In some countries, concentration of sodium hypochlorite solution is expressed in chloromatic degrees (0% Chloram); 1 chloram is approximately equivalent to 0.0% available chlorine (See Table 11.2).

The amount of available chlorine required in solutions for high-level infection depends on the amount of organic matter present, since chlorine is inactive by organic matter such as blood and pus.

Methods of Chemical Disinfection (Table 11.3)

- Immersion in high-level disinfectant for 30 minutes in a appropriate container
- Disinfections by wiping the exterior with a chemical. Wiping with an appropriate disinfectant is acceptable for surface such as table tops and for blood spills.

Aprons

Eye protection: Visors, goggles, safety spectacles should be worn whenever splashing body fluids or flying contaminated tissue expected.

Masks

Water repellant mask for blood splash to the face.

Sharps

Take care in using and disposing sharps. Do not resheathe sharps. Dispose in approved sharp container after breaking.

Table 11.2: Amount of chlorine in solutions for high-level infection

Material	*% of available chlorine*
Household liquid bleach	4.5%
Calcium liquid bleach	70%
Chlorinated lime	35%
NaDCC	60%
Chloramines	25%

Table 11.3: Strength of disinfectants used for disinfection

1.	Dettol	Chloroxylenol	1:20 to 1:100	Hand lotion, linen, utensils
2.	Hibitane	Chlorhexidine	1:100	Skin, instruments
3.	Eusol	Chlorine in the form of hypochlorite solution	1:80	Dressing, irrigation, storage, disinfection
4.	Cetrimide	Cetyl trimethyl ammonium bromide	1:100	Skin, utensils
5.	Lysol	Cresol and soap solution	1:40 to 1:80	Linen, floor
6.	Bradosol	Domiphen bormide	1:500	Utensils, linen, wound
7.	Savlon	0.3% chlorhexidine, 3% cetrimide	1:20 to 1:40	Equipment, trolleys, skin
8.	Phenol	Carbolic acid	1:10 to 1:20	Sanitary utensils, floor, excreta, linen, waste
9.	Sudol	50% phenol	1:10 to 1:20	Sanitary utensils, floor, excreta, linen, waste
10.	Formation	Formaldehyde water	50 gm/L of water for spray	Books, leather, rooms
11.	Panaform tablets	Formaldehyde	1:2	Elastic articles, endoscopes
12.	Cidex	Formaldehyde + Borax + Phenol	1:2	Surgical instrument
13.	Betadine	Iodine	1:40	Skin
14.	H_2O_2	Liberates O_2	1:80	Irrigation with warm water

Needlestick Injury

Encourage bleeding from wound. Do not suck or rub. Wash with soap and water. Cover with waterproof dressing. If known, note the name of patient. If patient is known for HIV, postexposure prophylaxis is necessary.

Spillage

Wear apron and gloves. Absorb liquid with paper towels. Put 1% hypochlorite solution or sprinkle sodium dichloroisocyanurate (NaDCC) granules and wait for 10 minutes. Clean with soap and water, discard articles in yellow bags.

Waste

All waste contaminated with blood or body fluids must be discarded in to yellow clinical waste sack bags and labeled and sent for incineration.

Transportation of Infected Patients

Before transferring client to wheelchair or stretcher, he is given clean gown to serve as robes.

Client with airborne route transmission should wear mask. Person accompanying may also wear barrier protection as needed.

Sometimes while transporting, client may drain body fluids onto stretcher or wheelchair. Ensure that equipment is cleaned after the client returns to the room. Extra sheet may be used to cover the stretcher or wheelchair seat.

Client on respiratory isolation is given tissues and bag to allow proper disposal of secretions. Nurse records type of isolation on chart.

Transmission Based Precautions

Airborne	Private room
Transmission measles, chickenpox, pulm TB	Negative pressure airflow and exchange/hair mask
Droplet	Private room, mask
Diphtheria	
Rubella	
Streptococcal pharaohs	
Pneumonia	
Scarlet fever	
Pertussis	
Mumps	
Sepsis	
P. plague	
Contact precautions	Private room gloves, gown
Respiratory virus	
Shigella	
Enterovirus	

Contd...

Contd...

Wound infections
Herpes simplex
Scabies

BIOMEDICAL WASTE MANAGEMENT

Definition

According to biomedical waste rules 1998 of India, "Biomedical waste" means any waste which is generated during the diagnosis, treatment, or immunization of human beings or animals or in research activities pertaining there to or in the production or testing of biological and including categories 1 to 10 specified.

Category 1	Human anatomical waste
Category 2	Animal waste
Category 3	Microbiology and biotechnology waste
Category 4	Waste sharps
Category 5	Discarded medicines and cytotoxic drugs
Category 6	Solid waste contaminated with blood and fluids
Category 7	Solid waste—Disposables, e.g. tubing, IV sets, catheter
Category 8	Liquid waste—Washing, cleaning
Category 9	Incineration ash
Category 10	Chemical used in production of biologicals, disinfectants and insecticides

Types of Hospital Waste

There are infectious, pathological, sharps, pharmacological, genotoxic, chemical, and radioactive wastes.

Category 1	Human tissues, organs, body parts
Category 2	
Category 3	Microbiology waste
Category 4	Waste sharps needles, scalpels, blades, glass which may cause puncture and cuts. It includes both used and unused sharps

Contd...

Contd...

Category 5	Discarded medicine and cytotoxic drugs
Category 6	Solid waste—Items contaminated with blood and body fluids—cotton gauge, dressings, plaster casts, linen, bedding, other material contaminated with blood, gown
Category 7	Solid waste—Tubings, catheters, IV sets, gloves
Category 8	Liquid waste—Waste generate from washing, cleaning
Category 9	Incineration ash

Average Composition of Hospital Waste in India

Glass	4%	Material	Percentage
General waste food, sweeping	53.5%	Paper	15%
		Plastics	10%
		Rags	15%
		Metals sharps	1%
		Infectious waste	1.5%

Hazards Associated with Hospital Waste

Exposure to hospital waste can result in disease or injury due to one or more following characteristics:

- It contains infectious agent
- It contains toxic and hazardous chemicals or pharmaceuticals
- It contains sharps
- It is genotoxic and radioactive.

All individuals exposed to such healthcare waste are potentially at risk those who generate waste and either handle or exposed to careless management.

- Pathogens in infectious waste may enter human body through puncture, abrasion or cut in the skin, through inhalation or ingestion. HIV hepatitis B, C, virus particularly may enter. Bacterias resistant to antibiotics and chemical disinfectants may also create hazards, if waste managed poorly
- Many chemicals and pharmaceuticals used are toxic, genotoxic, corrosive, inflammable, reactive, explosive or shock sensitive. They may cause burns, injury, intoxication
- Inhalation of dust, ingestion of food accidentally contaminated with cytotoxic drug

Table 11.4: Segregation of different types of waste

Color coding	*Type of container*	*Waste category*	*Treatment*
Yellow	Plastic bag	Cat. 1, 2, 3, 6	Incineration, deep burial
Red	Disinfected contained or plastic bag	Cat. 3, 6, 7	Autoclaving, microwaving chemical treatment, destruction, shredding
Blue/ White translucent	Plastic bag, puncture-proof container	Cat. 4, 7	Autoclaving, microwaving chemical treatment, destruction, shredding
Black	Plastic bag	Cat. 5, 9, 10 (Solid)	Disposal in secured land, fill

- Radioactive waste may cause headache, dizziness, vomiting and other serious problem.

Segregation, Transportation and Disposal

Segregation of different types of waste into different categories according to their treatment/disposal options (Table 11.4).

Chemical Treatment—1% Hypochlorite Solution

Mutilation and shredding to prevent reuse of waste collection bags for waste needing incineration shall not be made of chlorinated plastics.

- **Incineration:** It is high temperature dry oxidation process that reduces organic and combustible waste to inorganic incombustible matter and reduces volume and weight
- **Chemical disinfection:** Used for liquid waste like blood, urine, stool, sewage. Chemicals are added to waste to kill or inactivate the pathogens it contains
- **Screw feed technology:** It is non burn, dry thermal disinfection process in which waste is shredded and heated in rotating auger
- **Microwave irradiation:** Microwave of a frequency of 2450 MHz and wave length of 12.24 cm
- **Land disposal:** Open dumps and land fills.

CHAPTER

12

Administration of Medications

AIM

Students are able to administer, store drugs and take necessary precautions and the responsibility.

OBJECTIVES

- Students know weights and measures to administer drugs, prepare solutions
- Students know various abbreviations used in prescription and drug administrations
- Students know and are able to calculate the doses, dilution and prepare solutions
- Students understand nature and sources of drugs
- Students know different routes of drug administration
- Students understand policies regarding drug administration
- Students know and are able to take care of medicine cabinet and precautions in use and storage of dangerous drugs
- Students understand nurses responsibility in understanding prescription, administering drug, records and reports related to drug administration.

GENERAL PRINCIPLES: CONSIDERATIONS

Purpose of Medications

- To prevent, diagnose and treat disease
- To restore and maintain health

- To relieve pain and discomfort
- To produce analgesia and anesthesia
- To destroy pathogens and toxins in disease conditions
- To maintain blood glucose level
- To maintain normal blood pressure in hypertension
- To improve functions of vital organs
- To maintain normal physiology of the body
- To relieve congestion and pressure
- To maintain hormonal balance.

Nurses Responsibilities in Understanding Prescription, Administration of Drugs, Reports and Records in Relation to Drug Administration

Accountability and responsibility, nurse accepts the responsibility of all actions which includes administration of medicine. It is her responsibility to confirm that medicine does not do harm to patient. She must know therapeutic effect, usual dosage, side effects of all the medicines. She is responsible to ensure, clients who will self-administer medicines have been properly informed. Client receiving inappropriate medicine or failing to receive appropriate medicine is medication error. Preventing medication error is her responsibility. If occurs, it should be reported immediately to appropriate person. Right medication, right client, right dose, right route at right time to ensure safe medication, she should be aware of above five rights, a nursing standard of medication administration.

- Check the doctor's orders, prescription
- Compare the medications first ordered
- Check the label of medication three times, before removing from drawer or shelf, amount of medication when drawn from container and returning container to storage. When unit dosed prepacked containers are used, check with the medication form as it is not returned to storage.

Nurse who administers medication is responsible for its action/effects. Alert patient will know whether different medicine is offered and if he ask any questions not to ignore them as it may reveal error. Patients taking self-medication should keep them in original labeled container to avoid confusion. When medicines are prepared from larger source or strength then needed dose is to be calculated and measured with standard device. Tablet can be cut with knife, if half tablet is to be given. It also can be crushed with crushing device which is cleaned before and after. It should be mixed with very small amount of liquid or food. Favorite liquids of client may not be used as it may alter its taste and decreases the desire of patient for those liquids or foods. To identify right patient, check medication form against patients identity and ask patient his name in full. Consult the doctor, if you are unsure about the route and prescribed route is not recommended, consult immediately. Parenteral use medicines are labeled as for parenteral use only.

Table 12.1: Forms of drugs and its administration

Drug form		*Route of administration*
Caplet	-	Shaped like capsule and coated for easy swallowing
Capsule	-	Medication in powder form, liquid, oil and encased in gelatin shell
Elixir		Clear fluid containing water or/and alcohol
Extract	-	Concentrated medication form
Glycerite	-	Solution, medication combined with glycerin for external use, 50% glycerin
Intraocular disk	-	Small flexible, oval two soft outer layers and middle layer containing medication
Paste liniment	-	Preparation containing alcohol, oil or soapy emollient applied to skin
Lotion	-	Medication in liquid suspension applied externally
Solution	-	Liquid preparation used orally, parenterally, externally or instilled into body organ or cavity, water with dissolved compounds
Suppository	-	Solid dosage form mixed with gelatin and shaped in form of pellet for insertion into body cavity
Suspension	-	Finely divided drug particles, dispersed in liquid medium
Syrup	-	Medication dissolved in concentrated sugar solution
Tablet	-	Powdered dosage form compressed into hard disk or cylinder
Tincture	-	Alcohol or water alcohol medication
Transdermal disk or patch	-	Medication contained within semipermeable membrane or disk
Troche (Lozenges)	-	Flat, round containing medication, sugar and mucilage
Pill	-	Solid dosage form containing one or more medication shaped into globules, ovoid or oblong

ROUTES OF ADMINISTRATION (TABLE 12.1)

Oral Route

Easiest and most commonly used. Tablets, capsules are given by mouth and swallowed with water. Onset of action is slow and more prolonged than parenteral medications. Patient prefer oral route.

Sublingual Route

Some drugs are readily absorbed, if placed under tongue. They are not to be swallowed otherwise they will not effect, e.g. nitroglycerin. Until medicine is completely dissolved patient should not drink.

Buccal Route

Placing a solid medication in the mouth and against the mucous membrane of cheek until it dissolves.

Parenteral Routes

It is injecting a medication into body tissues.

- Subcutaneous - Below dermis of skin
- Intramuscular - Into muscle
- Intravenous - Into vein
- Intradermal - Into dermis under epidermis
- Epidural - Into epidural space via catheter
- Intrathecal - Into subarachnoid space via catheter or needle
- Intraosseous - Infusion into bone marrow
- Intrapleural - Into pleural space through chest wall
- Intra arterial - Into arteries
- Intra-articular - Into joint
- Inunction - Applying on skin and mucous membrane.
- Topical application - Moist dressings, soaking body parts in solution. Glycerine magnesium sulphate dressings.
- Instillation - Instilling fluid into body cavity, e.g. eardrops, eyedrops, nasal drops
- Topical application - Transdermal disk or patch, irrigation. Suppository, spraying
- Inhalation - From nose, mouth through tracheal tube.

STORAGE AND MAINTENANCE OF DRUGS

Drugs should be stored in cool, dry place away from patients reach and sunlight, free from dirt, cockroaches. Drugs are to be kept in safe place under lock and key. Tablets, capsules, pills should be kept in the same pack but if removed, than to be kept in clean bottle and labeled. Disinfectants, antiseptics are to be stored separately from medicines, which are digested or injected. Proper labeling is mandatory. Drugs are to be checked for their expiry date and are to be used before they are expired. Record of medicine indented, issued to patients is to be kept. Accounting of the drugs used should be done daily, weekly and monthly. Drugs which are prescribed most should be indented in more quantity depending on the requirement of patients in wards. Too many drugs which are not required should not be indented or are to be returned to the store before their expiry date. Account of dangerous drug is kept separately entering patient name, registration number, dose and total amount of drug used.

Broad Classification of Drugs

Analgesics	-	Drugs relieving pain
Antipyretic	-	Drugs reducing pyrexia
Anthelmintic	-	Antiworm infestation drugs
Antacids	-	Drugs neutralizing gastric acid
Antihypertensive	-	Drugs reducing blood pressure
Diuretic	-	Drugs increasing urine output
Sedatives	-	Drugs producing sleep
Tranquilizers	-	Drugs relieving anxiety
Antibiotics	-	Antibacterial or microbial
Antihistaminic	-	Drugs neutralizing histamines (allergens)
Expectorants	-	Drugs helping to bring out bronchial secretions
Cardiac stimulants	-	Drugs stimulating cardiac contractions
Respiratory stimulants	-	Drugs stimulating respiratory center
Hypoglycemic	-	Drugs reducing blood sugar level
Anti-inflammatory	-	Drugs reducing inflammatory process
Antiemetics	-	Drugs against vomiting
Bronchodilators	-	Drugs dilating bronchi
Anticonvulsions	-	Drugs preventing convulsions
Narcotics	-	Drugs producing sleep
Aperients	-	Drug producing action of bowels, a laxative
Antispasmodic	-	Drugs preventing muscle spasm

Effect of Drug Actions

Therapeutic effect, side effects, toxic effects, idiosyncratic reactions, allergic reactions, drug tolerance and drug interactions.

Therapeutic Effect

It is expected physiological response of medication, e.g. heparin is administered to dissolve thrombus. Aspirin is analgesic, antipyretic and anti-inflammatory and it reduces platelet aggregation.

Side Effects

These are unintended secondary effects that medicine predictably will cause. For example nausea, vomiting, black stools, irritation, etc.

Toxic Effect

Effects due to accumulation of drug or prolonged intake or excess dose. Opoids cause respiratory depression. Some drugs affect kidney function, heart function.

Idiosyncratic Reaction

It is unpredictable effects in which patient overact or under reacts to a medicine. Patient may have different reaction from normal, e.g. child may be excited after receiving Benadryl for allergy instead of feeling drowsy.

Allergic Reactions

These are unpredictable reactions in response to medicine. Patient may be sensitized to the first dose and later on develop allergic symptom after repeated doses of medicine, preservative or chemical acts as antigen and antibodies are released. Anaphylactic reactions, shock also may result. Mild allergic reactions are urticaria, rash, pruritus, rhinitis.

Drug tolerance and Drug Interactions

When one medication modifies the action of another medication, a medication interaction occurs. If several medications are taken together, drug interaction occurs.

Factors Influencing Drug Action

- Absorption
- Distribution
- Metabolism
- Excretion.

Constant therapeutic concentration is achieved by repeated doses because portion of medicine is excreted. Peak concentration is just before the last portion of medication, then the concentration falls progressively.

In intravenous infusion, peak concentration occurs immediately but falls quickly in serum level.

Drug Concentration: The point at which the lowest amount of drug is detected in the serum.

Serum half-life: Time taken to excrete to lower the serum level to half.

Therapeutic plateau: To maintain this, patient must receive regular fixed doses.

Oral medication have slow onset of action and more prolonged effect.

Some medicines are readily absorbed after being placed under the tongue. It should not be swallowed. Some are given by buccal route absorbed through buccal mucous membrane. Parenteral route involves injecting medicine into body tissue, body cavities, into vein, action may be local or systemic. Instillation of drops, inhalations, injection into spinal canal, epidural route will give local effects like regional and spinal anesthesia, anti-inflammatory action.

POLICIES IN RELATION TO DRUG ADMINISTRATION

Standing orders: Order is carried out till prescriber cancels it by another order or until prescribed number of days.

PRN orders: Prescriber orders when patient requires it.

Stat orders: Single dose of medication immediately or only once.

Prescription: It includes detailed information which patient can understand and follow.

Standing order is a document containing orders for the conduct of routine therapies, monitoring guidelines and diagnostic procedures for specific clients with identified clinical problems. Standing orders are approved and signed by the physician, in charge of care before their implementation. Standing orders and protocols give the nurses legal protection to intervene appropriately in the client's best interest.

Abbreviations

Abbreviations		*Meanings*
Ac	ac	before meals
ad lib		As desired
BID	bid, bd	Twice a day
h		hour
Hs	Hs	hour of sleep
PC	Pc	After meals
Prn		When needed
qarn		every morning
qd	OD	every day
QID	Qid	4 times a day
qh		every hour
q2h		every 2 hours
q4h		every 4 hours
q6h		every 6 hours
q8h		every 8 hours
STAT	stat	Give immediately
tid		Three times a day

System of Drug Measurements

Weights and Measures

Metric system is most logically organized. Metric units can easily be converted and computed through simple multiplication and division. Each basic unit is divided into 10 units multiplying or divided by 10 times secondary unit.

In multiplication, decimal point moves to right and in division to the left.

10.0 mg × 10 = 100 mg

10.0 mg × 10 = 0.1 mg

Meter—to measure length

Liter—to measure volume

Gram—to measure weight

Latin			Greek		
Deci	-	0. 1, 1/10	Deca	-	10
Centi	-	0. 01, 1/100	Hecto	-	100
Milli	-	0. 001, 1/1000	Kilo	-	1000

While writing doses, use metric system. For example, 500 mg or 0.5 g. 10 mL or 0.01 L.

Household Measurements

1 mL	-	15 drops gtt (gutta)
4–5 mL	-	1 teaspoon
16 mL	-	1 tablespoon
30 mL	-	2 tablespoon
240 mL	-	1 cup
480 mL	-	1 pint (pt)
960 mL	-	1 quart (qt)
3840 mL	-	1 gallon (gal)

Calculation of Doses, Preparation of Solutions

Solutions are used for:
- Injections
- Irrigations
- Infusions
- Topical applications.

Solutions is given mass of solid substance dissolved in a known volume of fluid or given volume of liquid dissolved in a known volume of another fluid.

When Solid is Dissolved in Fluid:
- Concentration is in units of mass per units of volume (9/mL, 9/L, mg/mL)
- Concentration of a solution may also be expressed as percentage. For example, 10 g of solid dissolved is 100 mL—10% can also be expressed as proportion. 1 g of solid dissolved in 1000 mL—1/1000. 1 mL of liquid dissolved in 1000 mL—1/1000.

Conversion within one system

Milligram to gram	Divide by 1000, moving 3 decimal points to the left
1000 mg-1 g	
250 mg-0.25 g	
1 L = 1000 mL	
0. 25 L = 250 mL	
Apothecary or household measurement	
1 qt = 32 ozs	8 dr = 10 g
8 ozs = 0. 25 qt or ¼ qt	1 dr = ¼ mL

1 tsf = 4 mL
1 tbsf = 15 mL
2 tbsf = 10 g = 30 mL

Dose Calculation

Dose ordered × amount = Amount to administer
Dose on hand, e.g. Demerol 50 mg is ordered
Medicine available in ampoule 100 mg/mL
Dose ordered—50 mg × amount on hand 1 mL = 0. 5 mL
Dose on hand—100 mg, e.g. Digoxin 0–125 mg, medicine available 0.25 mg
Dose ordered—0. 125 mg × 1 tablet = 0. 5
Dose on hand 0. 25 mg amount on hand
Dose order 250 mg, e.g. 5 mL contains 125 mg of erythromycin
250 mg × 5 mL = 10 mL to administration 125 mg.

Paratactic Doses

Surface area of child × normal adult dose 1.7 m^2
Weight 12 kg surface 0. 54 m^2 = 0. 3 mg
Area 1.7 m^2 × 250 mg = 75 mg

TECHNIQUES OF DRUG ADMINISTRATION

Oral

It is easiest and common route of drug administration. Medicines are given by mouth and swallowed with fluid. They have slow onset of action and prolonged effect.

Sublingual

Medicines designed to use as sublingual are placed under the tongue. They are not swallowed. Nitroglycerine is commonly given by sublingual route. No drink is taken. Drug gets dissolved and absorbed.

Buccal

Medicine is placed in mouth against mucous membrane of cheek till it is dissolved. Use alternate cheek to prevent irritation. Client is warned not to chew or swallow it.

Equipment

Medicine cart or tray, disposable medicine cups, glass of water or juice, straw, pill crushing device, paper towels, order book or computer print out.

Procedure

- Assess for any contraindications, assess for any allergy
- Check laboratory data which may influence medication administration
- Assess patient's fluid preference
- Check accuracy and completeness of written order for medication—name, medicine, dose, route, time
- Wash hands. Prepare medicine. Arrange cups and medicine on cart or trolley
- Prepare medication for one patient at a time
- Select correct medication, check label, check order
- Calculate medication dose as needed. Double check calculations.

Topical Administration

Purpose

Relief of pain, smoothening, stimulate, reduce edema, irrigate/wash, reduce inflammation, stop hemorrhage, vasoconstriction, dilation or constriction of pupil, correct or prevent infection.

Sites

Skin, nose, eyes, ears, vagina, rectum and mouth.

Equipment

Skin: Lotion, paste, ointment, gloves, applicator.
Wound: Sterile articles, gloves, lotion, ointment, powder, glycerine magsulf, Vaseline gauze, whichever is ordered.
Nose: Nasal spray, drops, tampons, gloves, forceps.
Eye: Eyedrops, eye ointments, discs, artificial tears, vasoconstrictor eyedrops, mydriatics, miotics, saline swabs, tissues, paper bag, emesis basin.

Application to Skin

Medicines applied to the skin are in the form of lotions, pastes, ointments which can create systemic effect. Nurse should apply these medications using gloves or applicators. If wound is present use, aseptic technique. Spread the medication evenly. Gauze dressing is applied sometimes. Smearing, rubbing may cause irritation sometimes. Thin layer of powder is dusted some times. Record name of medication, area, and condition of the skin.

Application to Mucous Membrane

Gel and glycerine is applied to oral mucous membrane. If antifungal drops like candid or gentian violet is to be applied, put a drop of medicine on tongue. It spreads on oral mucous membrane.

Gargles

Saline, warm water, condy's lotion, other solutions used for mouth wash may be used for gargles diluted in water. Small amount of water or solution is taken in oral cavity and ask the patient to move the solution to all the parts without swallowing for 30 seconds and spit out.

Direct Application of Liquids

Some solutions are applied directly over the area with swabstick.

Insertion of Drug into Body Cavity: Suppositories

Vaginal and rectal suppositories are available. They are wrapped in foil and stored in refrigerator. Body temperature causes it to melt when placed in vagina. Rectal suppositories are thinner and more bullet-shaped with rounded end to prevent anal trauma during insertion. Vaginal foam, tablets, jellies, and cream are administered with an applicator, inserter. With gloved hand, suppositories are inserted with aseptic technique. Client can self-introduce suppository. Privacy is to be provided. Rectum should be empty before insertion of it. It is to be placed beyond internal sphincter or else it is expelled easily.

Medicated Packing in Rectum

Acriflavine, glycerine magsulf pack may be inserted after operation on rectum, colon. Sloughing wounds, foul smelling discharge, may need packing of rectum for few hours and solutions used are acriflavine, betadine.

Medicated Packing in Vagina

Vagina may be temporarily packed with long strip of sterile gauze to control bleeding. Tampon are placed while repairing perineum. Packing may be done after operations on vagina, cervix for few hours.

Instillation

Eye

Cornea is very sensitive to anything applied to it. Avoid any drop or ointment application directly on it. Avoid touching eye structures with eye droppers, ointment tubes, to prevent cross infection to other eye. Never allow client to use other patient's eye medicine. Some medicines are administered intraocularly. It remains in conjunctival sac for a week. It is like contact lense. Pilocarpine is administered in this way.

Ear

Any drops, irrigation solution should be at room temperature. No force should be used. Ensure ear drum is intact. Straighten the ear canal by holding auricle, and gently pulling down and backward.

CHAPTER 13

Meeting the Needs of Perioperative Patients (Preoperative, Intraoperative and Postoperative)

AIM

Students give care to clients preoperatively and postoperatively and during the operation.

OBJECTIVES

- Students are able to define three phases of perioperative period
- Explain the process of wound healing
- Describe the principles and techniques of wound care
- Perform care of wounds.

Definition and concept of perioperative nursing management during a period of time that constitutes the surgical experience, include preoperative, intraoperative and postoperative phases of nursing care.

Elective or emergency surgery is stressful and even complex. Advance surgical techniques, anesthesia, and many surgical procedures nowadays can be performed in ambulatory setting.

Hospital stay for operation is decreased. Many patients are admitted for operation the same day morning and discharged in the evening. Hospital stay is required for trauma patients, acutely ill patients, major surgeries, emergency surgery and patients with concurrent medical disorder.

Today operations such as microsurgery, laser surgery, laparoscopic surgery, bypass surgery, organ transplant require monitoring.

Newer drugs for anesthesia and pain management are of help and reduce the postoperative nausea, vomiting and shorten the time of recovery.

Preadmission testing, preoperative preparation, competent ambulatory care, same day surgery, patient care requires sound knowledge of all the aspects of preoperative care.

PREOPERATIVE PHASE

Preoperative phase begins when operation is decided and ends when the patient reaches operation room table.

Preparation of a Patient for Surgery

- Establishing baseline evaluation of the patient before the day of surgery by carrying out preoperative interview, includes:
  - Physical and emotional assessment
  - Previous anesthetic history
  - Identification of known allergies, genetic problem
  - Preadmission tests
  - Appropriate consultative service
  - Preparatory education about recovery from anesthesia and post-operative care.
- Review of the patients teaching on the day of surgery, verification of the patients identity, surgical sites, confirm informed consent, starting intravenous infusion. Verifying for safe transport availability and person to accompany, if patient is discharged the same day
- Updating preoperative patient assessment addressing to the queries of patient and family
- Verifying preoperative orders by the surgeon
- Assess the risk for postoperative complications
- Report unexpected findings or any deviation from normal
- Assess patient's status, review charts, identify patient, verify surgical site, administer medicine, ensure contact, provide psychological support. Communicate patient's emotional status to other appropriate members of the healthcare team
- Blood tests, X-rays and other diagnostic tests are performed, when indicated, through physical assessment and history
- Optimum nutrition for promoting healing. Correction of malnutrition
- Correction of thirst and electrolyte deficit
- A person with history of chronic alcoholism suffers from malnutrition and other systemic problems may increase the risk. Care is necessary before planning for surgery.

- Optimum respiratory function is required. Patient is taught deep breathing exercise and use of incentive spirometer
- Patients with respiratory diseases are assessed carefully and smoking is stopped at least 24 hours before the surgery
- Cardiopulmonary function is ensured. Surgery may be postponed till blood pressure is under control
- Urinary output should be normal
- A patient with diabetes undergoing surgery, is at risk of hyper- and hypoglycemia and acidosis. Blood sugar level is important before, during and after surgery
- Use of corticosteroid during preceding year must be reported to anesthetist and surgeon, as there is risk of adrenal insufficiency
- Determine existence of allergies
- Any medication, if patient is using in the past is to be documented and informed
- Preoperative anxiety may be due to threat to his role in life, body integrity, or life itself. Identify any anxiety patient is experiencing
- Make an attempt to provide spiritual help. Faith has great sustaining power. Belief of each patient should be respected and supported
- Attention to be paid to patient with special considerations, e.g. ambulatory surgery, geriatric patient, obese and disabled
- Quick visual survey for trauma patients when emergency surgery is needed.

Immediate Preoperative Nursing Interventions

- Withholding food and fluid at least 8 hours before surgery
- Preparing bowel for surgery—enema is ordered for patients undergoing abdominal and pelvic surgery. Laxative may be ordered previous night
- Preoperative skin preparation—use soap containing germicide for several days before surgery to reduce the number of organisms. Hair at or around the incision site are removed
- Hospital gown is provided. Long hair are braided, remove hairpins and cover head completely with disposable paper cap or cloth

  Mouth is inspected, dentures and plates are removed. Jewelery is removed and valuables are given to family members or labeled clearly and stored in the safe place
- All the patients, except those with urological disorder, should void before going to operation room

- Urinary catheterization may be performed, if necessary
- Preanesthetic medicine is given. Patient is kept in bed with side rails and observed. Premedication is given many times when called for operation as the schedule may change or operation is delayed
- Completed checklist of preoperative check accompanies the patient with surgical consent form attached along with laboratory reports and nurses records
- The patient is transferred to holding area 30 minutes before the anesthetic is to be given, on stretcher with small head pillow and blanket
- The patient is greeted by name, positioned comfortably on bed or stretcher
- Varification of the patient, site of operation and surgical procedures is for patients safety.

INTRAOPERATIVE PHASE

Operation Theater Setup and Environment

- Stark appearance, cool temperature, double doors, restricted entry, surgical asepsis, health of staff, cleanliness of rooms, sterility of equipment and surfaces, processes of scrubbing, gowning (Fig. 13.1).
- Located central to supportive services such as pathology, radiology, laboratory, special air filtration device. Control of humidity, temperature and airflow.
- Surgical area is divided into three zones—unrestricted zone, semi-restricted zone and restricted zone.
  - Unrestricted zone: Street clothes are allowed
  - Semi-restricted zone: Attire consists of gown, mask and caps
  - Restricted zone: Scrub clothes, shoe covers, caps and masks are worn.

Surgeon and surgical team wear additional sterile gown and protective device during operations.

Masks are worn all the time in restricted zone. It should fit snugly over nose and month (Fig. 13.2).

Head gear should completely cover the hair. Skin infections, sore throat, respiratory infection to be reported, surgical asepsis—all surgical supplies, any instrument, needles, sutures, dressings, gloves, covers, solutions must be sterilized before use.

Surgical team wear long-sleeved sterile gowns (Fig. 13.2), head and hair are covered with cap, mask is worn over the nose and mouth. Patient's skin

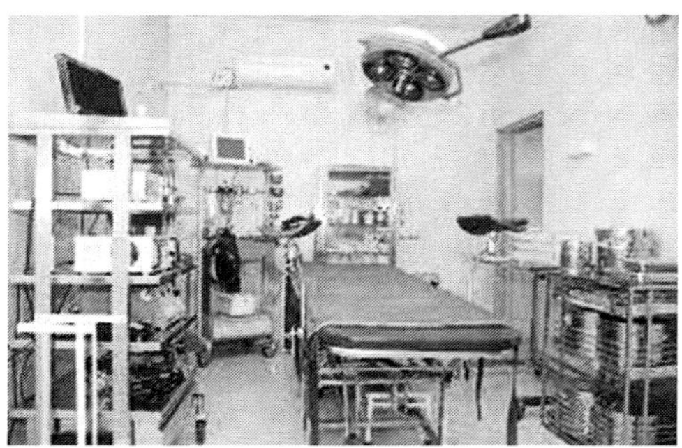

Fig. 13.1: Operation theater

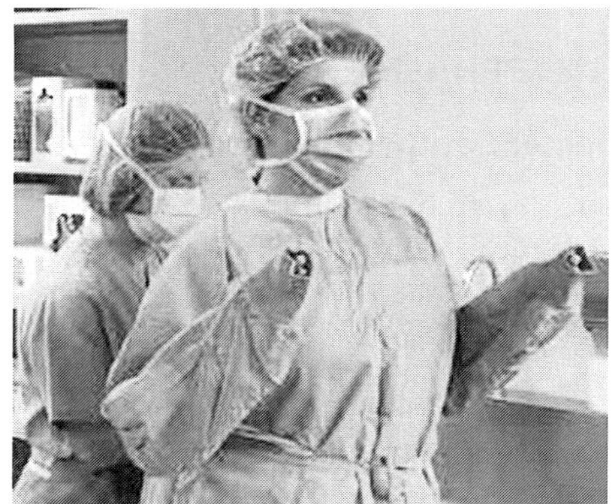

Fig. 13.2: Wearing mask, gown, head cover

is cleaned and antimicrobial is applied over the large area near incision site. Body is covered with sterile drapes.

Environment

Floors and horizontal surfaces are cleaned frequently with detergent, soap and water or detergent germicide. Sterilizing, e.g. equipment are inspected regularly to ensure the optimum functions.

All instruments are cleaned and sterilized in a unit near to operation room.

All equipment that comes in contact with the patient must be sterile.

Gowns of sterile team are considered sterile in front from chest to level of sterile field. Sterile drapes are used to create sterile field. Item should be dispensed to sterile field by methods that preserve the sterility of the item and integrity of the sterile field. Every sterile field should be constantly monitored and maintained.

For AIDS, addition of double gloves, goggles, waterproof aprons, sleeve protectors is necessary.

Anesthesia

Inhalation anesthesia or intravenous anesthesia is used for operations (General anesthesia).

Regional and spiral anesthesia is also used for many operations. Epidural anesthesia, brachial plexus block, paravertebral anesthesia and transpolar are the types of anesthesia used (Fig. 13.3).

Role of a Nurse

- Providing safety and well-being of the patient
- Coordinating with operating room personnel
- Performing scrub and circulating activities
- Continue the care begun by preoperative nurses care

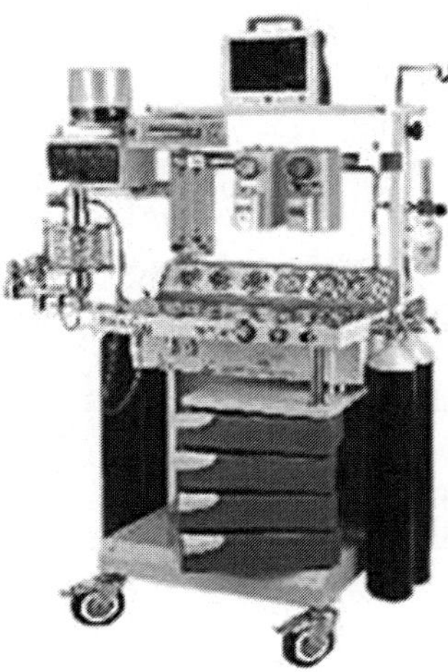

Fig. 13.3: Anesthesia trolley

- Reassure the patient and provide information
- Support the coping strategies and reinforce the patient's ability to influence the outcomes
- Encourage active participation in the plan of care
- Monitor factors that can cause injury such as patient's position, equipment malfunction, environmental hazards
- Protect the patient's dignity and interests when anesthetized
- Maintain existing patient risk factors
- Identify existing patient risk factors
- Assist in modifying complicating factors and reducing operating risk
- Circulator or circulating nurse must be a registered nurse and monitors activities of surgical team. Check operating room conditions. Assess patient for injury and inference.

Verify consent, ensure cleanliness, coordinate, maintain temperature, humidity, lighting, safe functioning of equipment, availability of supplies and materials.

Monitor aseptic practice and avoid breaks in technique. Monitor patient's condition.

Scrub Role

- Performing surgical hand scrubs (Figs 13.4 to 13.6)
- Setting up sterile tables (Figs 13.4A and B)
- Preparing sutures, ligatures, and special equipment, e.g. laparoscopes
- Assisting surgeon
- Surgical assistance during the surgery by anticipating instruments that will be required. Such as sponges, drains, other equipment
- As the incision is closed, scrub person and circular count all needles, sponges, instruments to be sure they are accounted for and not retained in the body of the patient
- Tissue specimens obtained during surgery must also be labeled by scrubbing nurse and sent to laboratory by circulator.

Registered Nurse First Assistant

- Handling tissues
- Providing exposure at operative field
- Suturing and providing hemostasis
- Handling emergencies
- Surgical asepsis.

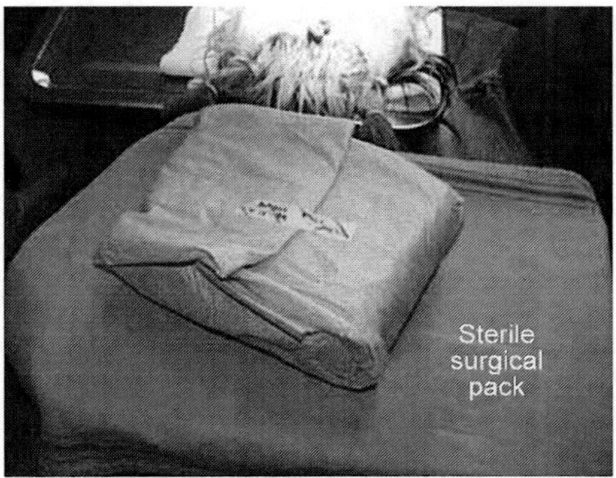

Fig. 13.4A: Opening sterile pack

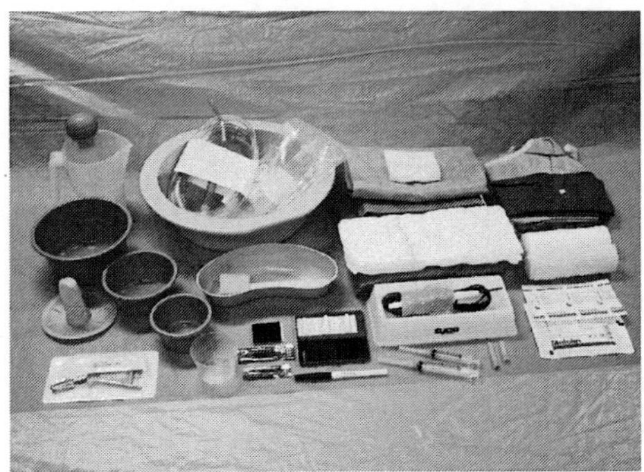

Fig. 13.4B: Opened sterile pack

POSTOPERATIVE PHASE

Recovery Unit—Postanesthesia Care Unit (PACU)

It is located adjacent to operating rooms. Patients still under anesthesia or recovering from anesthesia are placed in this unit.

It is to be kept clean, quiet away from unnecessary equipment, well-ventilated, light painted, with soundproof ceiling, isolated, out visible quarters for disrupted patients.

The PACU bed provides easy access to the patients, safe and easily movable, adjustable for change of position of the patient, provision to facilitate care such as IV poles, side rails, wheel brakes, and chest storage rack.

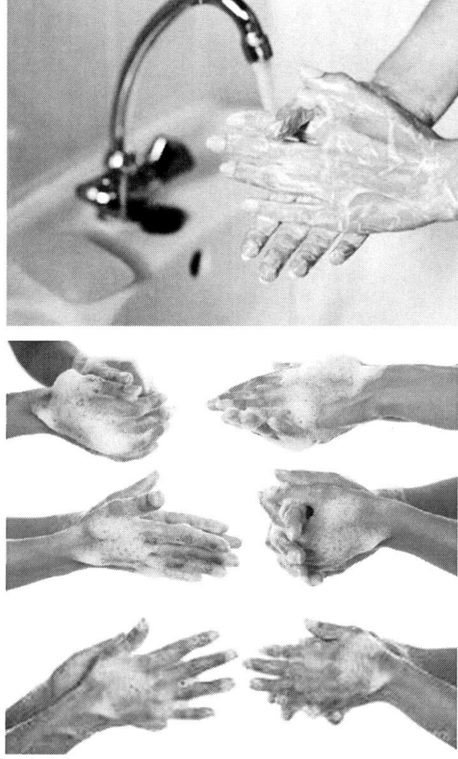

Fig. 13.5: Hand wash

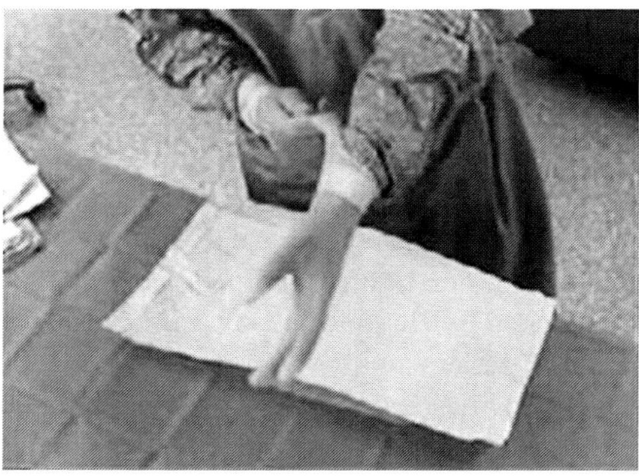

Fig. 13.6: Gloving

Postanesthetic Care

Phase I

Immediate recovery phase—needs intensive nursing care. Frequent monitoring of patient's pulse, electrocardiogram (ECG), respiratory rate, blood pressure and pulse oximeter value.

Keeping air passage patent, ready to reintubate, and handling other emergencies. Patient is transferred to PACU from OT by anesthetist. He accompanies the patient during transfer and remains at the head of the stretcher and maintains airway.

While transporting the patient, special attention to incision site, vascular changes, and exposure is paid so as to prevent strain and obstructing drains, IV infusion, change of position moving slowly and carefully; patient is placed on bed.

Gown is changed, if soiled, covered with blanket, side rails are raised.

Review diagnosis, surgery performed, age, general condition, airway patency, vital signs, medications and anesthetics used during surgery, problems occurred during procedure, pathology encountered, fluid administered, estimated blood loss and fluid replacement, tubings and drains, catheters or supportive aids.

- Frequent skilled assessment of blood oxygen saturation level, pulse rate, rhythm, depth and nature of respiration, skin color, level of consciousness
- Check surgical site for drainage and hemorrhage, connected drainages are functioning
- Monitor vital signs every 15 minutes
- Observe for choking, noisy breathing, movement of chest and diaphragm, exaled breath, cyanosis
- Do not remove airway till gag reflex is seen
- Cautious suctioning, turn the patient's head to one side, elevation of head 15–30°, helps to maintain airway
- If vomiting occurs, turn the patient's head and collect vomitus in emesis basin, suction the pharynx with catheter tip.

Phase II

The patient requires less frequent observation and prepared to transfer to postoperative unit. The patient may remain for 4–6 hours depending on the type of surgery and pre-existing condition of the patient. Nurses working in PACU have special skills.

Postoperative Care

Seriously ill patients, patients with major cardiovascular, pulmonary or neurosurgery are admitted to special intensive care units.

For patients returning to general surgical wards after surgery, room is prepared assembling necessary equipment and supplies like IV pole, drainage receptor holder, emesis basin, tissues, disposable pads, blanket, charts and forms.

When patient is received from the recovery room, nurse from recovery room reports the baseline data and medications given, general condition of patient, events occurred, etc. to ward nurse. The receiving nurse reviews data, postoperative orders and attends patient's immediate needs.

Nursing Management

- Assess physiological status frequently
- Pain management: Assess pain level, administer ordered analgesic
- Management of therapeutic regimen
- Monitoring for complications
- Monitor temperature every 4 hours for 24 hours; pulse every 15 minutes for 1st hour; and every 30 min for 2 hours. Assess patency of IV line, administer appropriate fluids
- Observe spontaneous voiding, palpate bladder for fullness
- Deep breathing and leg exercise, elastic stockings
- Next day ambulation, light meal
- Turning frequently and taking deep breath every 2 hours
- Coughing is contraindicated in the patients with head injury or neurosurgery and eye surgery
- Incentive spirometer for the patients with thoracic and abdominal surgeries. Ten deep breaths every hour
- Encourage activity
- Hourly output is measured, if less than 30 mL/hr reported
- Electrolyte, hemoglobin and hematocrit are monitored
- Management of surgical drains and dressings
- Inspection of incision site for approximation of edges, integrity of sutures, redness, discoloration and warmth
- Allow the escape of blood and serious fluid drainage of these fluids by penrose, hemovac and Jackson Pratt drains
- Record wound drainage output

- Wound healing occurs in three phases—(i) inflammatory, (ii) proliferative and (iii) maturation and by 1st, 2nd or 3rd intention.
- If cyanoacrylate tissue adhesive is used to close incision without use of sutures, dressing is contraindicated
- Infected wounds heal by 2nd or 3rd intention. Healing is by granulation. It is packed with saline moistered dressings and covered with dry sterile dressing
- Its postoperative dressing is usually changed by the surgeon or assistant and subsequent dressings are done by the nurse
- Nurse carries out hand hygiene before and after dressing and wears disposable gloves. Pull the adhesive parallel to skin, wipe with alcohol to remove the adhesive. Old dressing is removed and put in container designated for biomedical waste disposal
- Teach the patient how to care for incision and change the dressing at home
- In postoperative patient suffering from abdominal distesion, results from accumulation of gas and can be prevented by change of position, ambulation, nasogastric aspiration. Document bowel sounds when starting oral fluids
- Laxative may be ordered, if constipation problem on 3rd day after operation.

Wound Healing

Wound: Break in the continuation of tissues or disruption in the continuity of cells.
Healing: Restoration of continuity.

Types of Wounds

Incised: Clean cut with sharp instrument, e.g. knife, scalps.
Confused: Made by blunt force.
Lacerated: Jagged, irregular edges, made by glass, wire, animal paws.
Punctured: They result in small opening in skin and wound is deep, e.g. gun shot, knife injury.
Clean wound: Surgical wounds.
Contaminated: Accidental, inflamed wounds.
Infected: Organisms are present before surgery or organisms entering from environment.

Phases of Wound Healing

Inflammatory Phase

When tissue is cut or injured, vascular and cellular response occurs immediately. Vasoconstriction and clot formation occurs to control bleeding (5–10 min).

Histamine is released increasing capillary permeability. Neutrophils move to damaged area. Macrophages engulf the debris and remove it from the area. Antigen and antibodies also appear. Basal cells at the wound edges undergo mitosis. Proteolytic enzymes are secreted and blood clots are dissolved. Gap meets usually within 24–48 hours. At this stage, cell migration is enhanced by hyperplastic bone marrow activity.

Proliferative Phase

Fibroblasts multiply and lattice framework is formed for migrating cells. Epithelial cells from edges of wound buds develop into capillaries which supply nutrition to granulation tissues.

Granulation Phase

Granulation tissue consisting of new capillary buds, phagocytes, fibroblasts develops invading the clot and restoring the blood supply to the wound. Fibroblasts continue to secrete collagen fibers as the clot and bacteria are removed by phagocytosis.

Maturation Phase

Granulation tissue is replaced by fibrous scar tissue. Rearrangement of collagen fibers occurs and the strength of the wound increases. In time, the scar becomes less vascular appearing after few months as fine line. The channels left when stitches are removed; heal by same process.

Secondary Healing

Healing by second intention—This method of healing follows distruction of large amount of tissue or when the edges of the wound cannot be brought into apposition, e.g. varicose ulcer, pressure ulcer. Stages are same as primary healing. Time taken depends on size of the wound and effective removal of the cause.

Fibrosis (Scar Formation)

Fibrous tissue is formed during healing by secondary intention, e.g. following chronic inflammation, persistent ischemia, suppuration or large trauma. Process begins with formation of granulation tissue, then overtime, the new capillaries and inflammatory material is removed leaving only collagen fibers secreted by fibroblasts. Fibrous tissue may have long-lasting damaging effect.

Complications

Adhesions, tissue shrinkage, infection and abscess.

Wound Dressing

Purpose

- To clean and dress the wound
- To prevent entry of microbes
- To protect the wound from harm and further injury
- To enhance healing process.

Equipment (Sterile)

- Sterile dressing packs may be kept in sterile drums (Fig. 13.7)
- Sterile tray
- Sterile gloves
- Sterile pack (Fig. 13.8)
- Sterile gauze pieces (folded)
- Cotton swabs. Sterile bowls (small)
- Artery forceps
- Dissecting forceps (Fig. 13.9)
- Cotton pad (Fig. 13.10)
- Bandage (Fig. 13.11A).

Tray (Cleaning)

- Disposable gloves
- Lotions: Betadine
- Antiseptic cream: Acriflavine
- Like soframycin: Mercurochrome

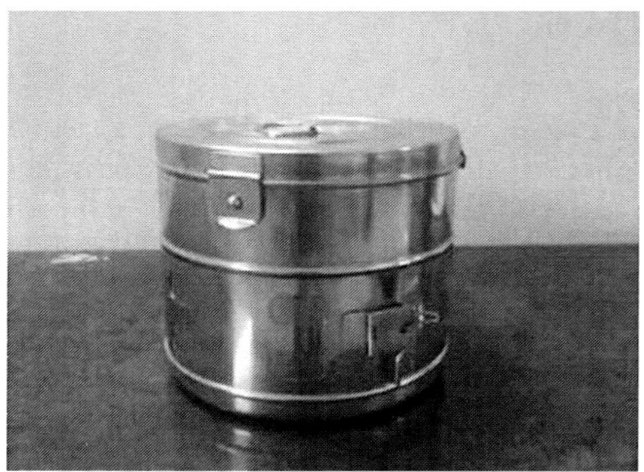

Fig. 13.7: Dressing drum

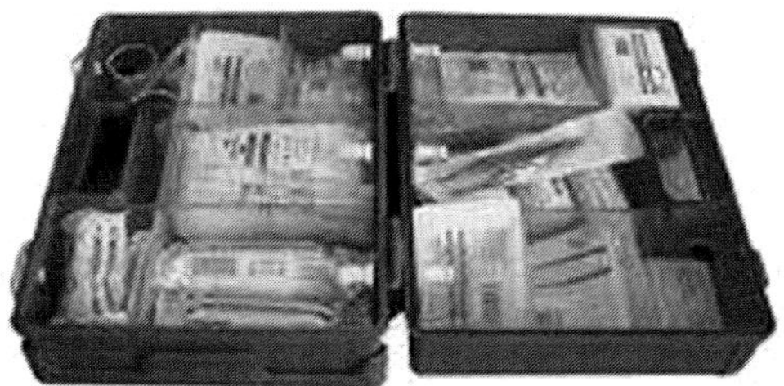

Fig. 13.8: Dressing pack

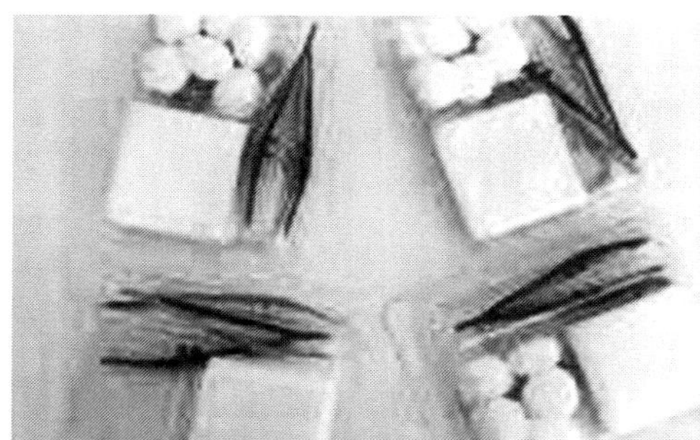

Fig. 13.9: Swab, forceps

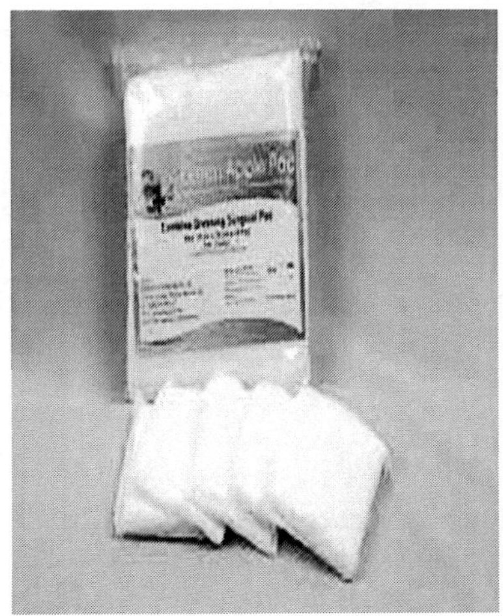

Fig. 13.10: Dressing

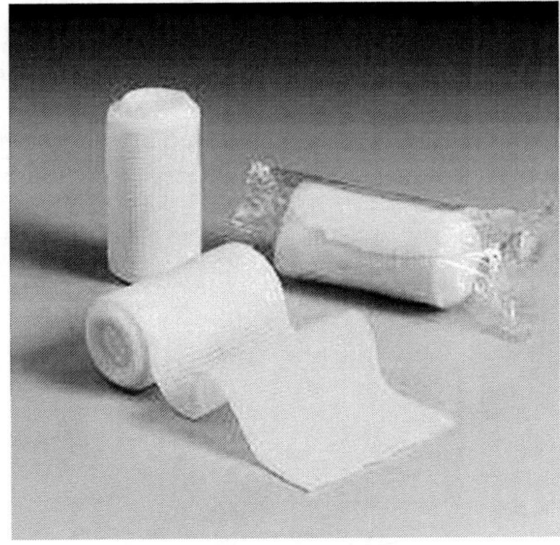

Fig. 13.11A: Bandage

- Neosporin: Spirit
- Glycerine Magsulf: Normal saline savlon
- Vaseline gauze: Adhesive plaster scissors.

Other Equipment

- Mackintosh
- Towel or draw sheet
- Kidney tray
- Paper bag.

Procedure

Explain the procedure to the client. Assemble all articles on a trolley either bring the client to dressing room or take dressing trolley (Fig. 13.11B) near client's bed. Screen the bed. Use proper lighting. If two nurses perform the dressing, it is better. One performs the dressing and the other assists.

- Wash hands, wear mask and gown
- Assistant can give the comfortable position and an access to the wound place mackintosh, towel under the part
- Loosen the dressing. If necessary, use adhesive remover. Place opened cuffed plastic bag nearby
- Use clean disposable gloves. Remove soiled dressing from the wound. Do not reach to wound. Discard the dressing in the bag. Remove gloves and discard.

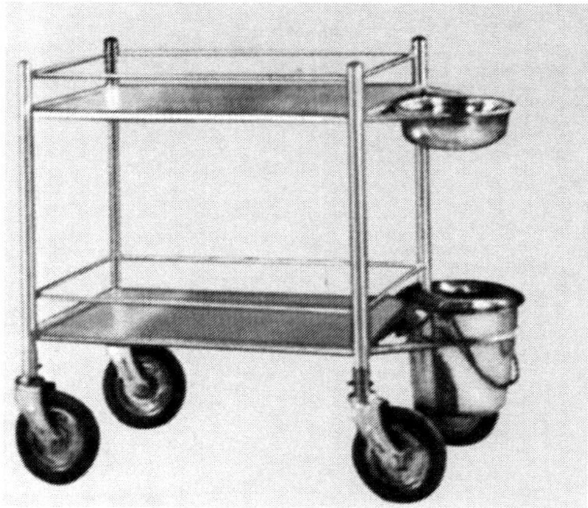

Fig. 13.11B: Dressing trolley

- Open dressing pack, containing bowls, cotton swabs, gauze
- Pour solution required in bowl over gauze piece
- Wear sterile gloves, observe wound. Clean the area around the wound from near the wound to periphery without touching the wound with savlon with cotton swab or gauze piece dipped in savlon, use 2–3 swabs. Clean wound area using another piece of gauze with savlon. Discard all swabs and gauze in paper bag kept in kidney tray
- Clean around the drain, if present
- Clean with normal saline swabs
- Dry the wound with dry gauze
- Apply antiseptic cream or powder as ordered. If powder used directly, it can be sprinkled over wound. If cream is used, apply on a layer of gauze or directly over the wound
- Apply sterile fold of gauze square
- Apply cotton pad
- Apply adhesive, if over abdomen
- Apply bandage, if on the other body areas
- Remove gloves after washing hands
- Remove mackintosh, towel underneath
- Discard paper bag containing swabs
- Keep trolley away
- Make the client comfortable
- Wash hands again with soap and water
- If wound is infected, the same trolley should not be used
- Clean wound, dressing is to be done first
- For infected wounds, other equipment are to be used and solutions which are used are eusol (for slough), glycerine magsulf
- Transparent film dressings which have one side adhesive can be used as primary dressing in the wounds where minimal tissue loss and less drainage is present. Hydrocolloidal dressings are made of gelling agents and have adhesive wound surface. Various sizes and shapes are available and are used to cover the wound 1–1.5" beyond the wound. Margin gel remains in contact with the wound and maintains moisture. It can be kept for several days
- Vacuum-assisted closure is the treatment for chronic wounds; open foam sponge is placed over the wound, sealed with transparent dressing and tube is placed over the wound within foam. Negative pressure in prescribed amount is created which removes excess fluid by suction.

Suture Care

Sutures are threads, wire—silk, steel, cotton, nylon, dacron. These are used to sew body tissues.

- **Skin sutures:** Steel staples, steristrips, dacron, linen, silk
- **Muscles and fascia:** Chromic catgut, plain catgut 0–2 no.

Sutures are placed within tissue layers in deep wounds and superficially for wound closure.

When dressing the wound, sutures are touched with spirit or betadine. When removing, check the type of sutures used, intermittent or continuous. Retention sutures are deeper than skin sutures and are not removed by the nurse. Never pull the visible portion through underlying tissue. Hold the suture material as close to the skin as possible.

Care of Drainage

- Drain must be placed in the dependent position, if gravity alone is to accomplish the drainage. Sump tube must be used to remove the drainage
- The drainage is brought out through the shortest route from abdominal wall to avoid kinking
- Proper dressing of drainage site daily to be done to prevent the infection
- Clean the tube with savlon swab or betadine swab
- Portex intercostal drainage tube should be connected to under water seal bottle by extension tubing. It is used to drain pleural cavity.

Bandaging

Purpose

- To apply pressure to stop hemorrhage
- To protect and secure dressings over wound
- To reduce edema
- To immobilize the part
- Securing splint
- To support large wounds.

Material used: Woven cotton, domette

Size: For fingers—1" or 2.5 cm

For hand—2" or 5 cm

For arm—2.5" or 7.5 cm

For breast—4 to 6" or 10–15 cm
For thighs—6" or 15 cm
For legs—4 to 6" or 10–15 cm
For head—2.5" or 7.5 cm.

Principles or Rules

- See that bandage is tightly rolled before attempting to use it
- Apply outer side of free end to the part
- Start from below and go upwards and from within outwards over the limb
- Cover the preceding layer 2/3rd with every turn
- Apply bandage firmly and evenly and not too tight or loose
- Fix with safety pin when finished
- Do not drop the bandage
- Wash hands before bandaging.

Methods

- **Simple spiral:** Encircling the part several times, used when part is of the same thickness, e.g. finger, wrist
- **Reverse spiral:** Bandage is reversed downwards upon itself at each term. This is used when thickness varies, e.g. Forearm, leg (Fig. 13.12)
- **Figure of 8:** Bandage is passed obliquely around the limb alternately upwards and downwards loops resembling 8. It is used near the joints, e.g. elbow, knee (Figs 13.13 to 13.15)
- **Spica:** It is modified figure of 8—used for 90° joints, e.g. shoulder groin, thumb (Figs 13.16 to 13.20)
- **Capeline (Figs 13.21 and 13.22):** For head, take 2½", 2 bandages and joint in the middle free ends. Stand behind the client, making him comfortable sitting in chair. Apply the joint to the middle of forehead just above the eyebrow. Bandage in the right hand is called vertical bandage and bandage in the left hand is called as horizontal. Bring both the rolls to back of the head and cross them (Fig. 13.22A). Carry vertical bandage forward over the head and horizontal bandage around the head and cover the vertical bandage in front; continue to pass the vertical bandage backwards and forwards each time little to the left and right alternately locking it with horizontal bandage (Fig. 13.22B). Finally, pass the horizontal bandage twice around the head and pin in front (Fig. 13.22C).

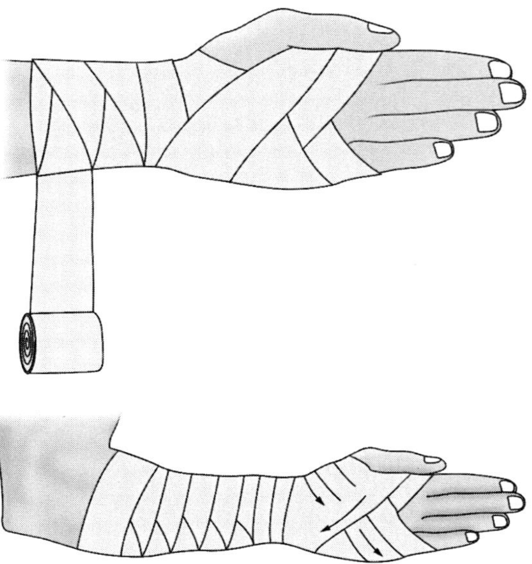

Fig. 13.12: Reverse spiral for forearm

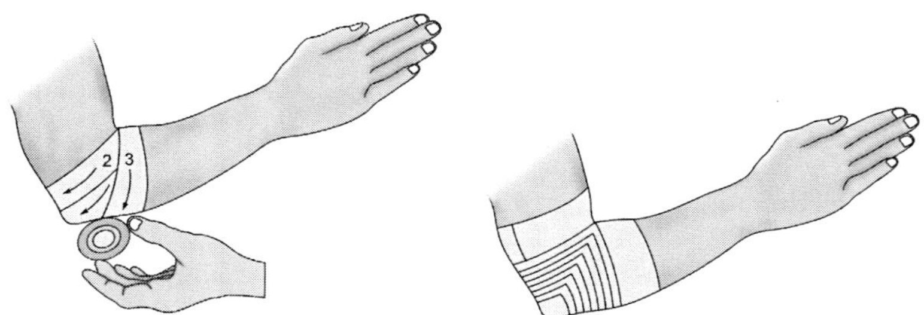

Fig. 13.13: Figure of 8 (Elbow, knee, ankle)

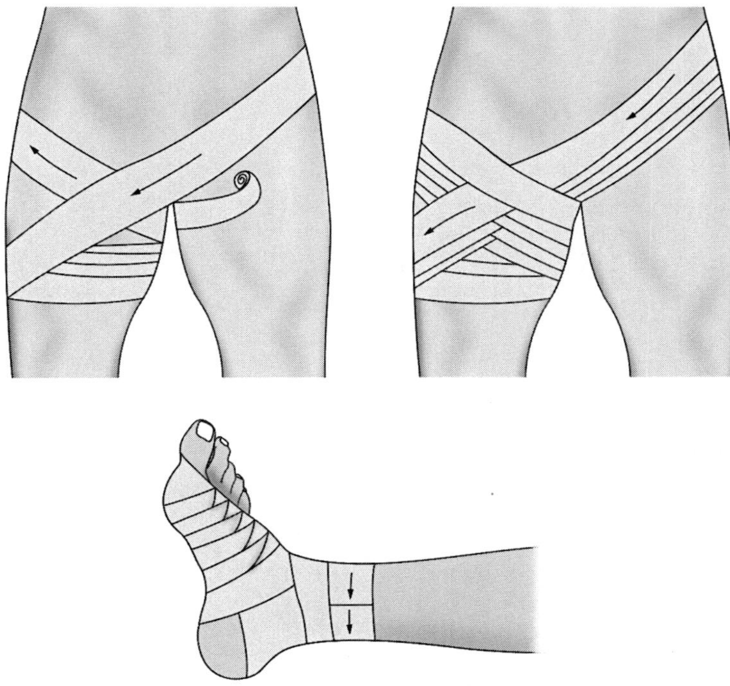

Fig. 13.14: Bandage for foot

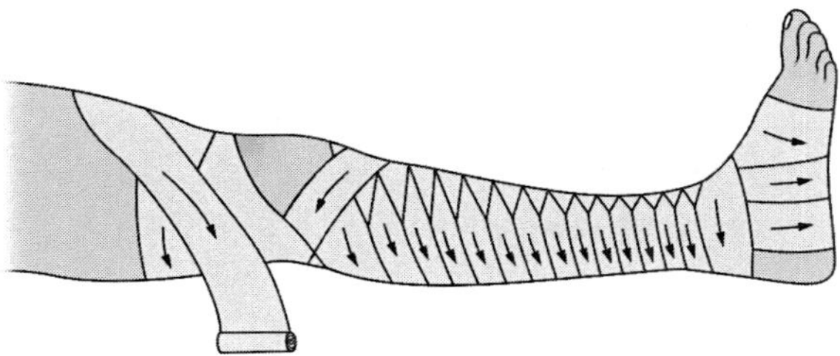

Fig. 13.15: Bandage for foot

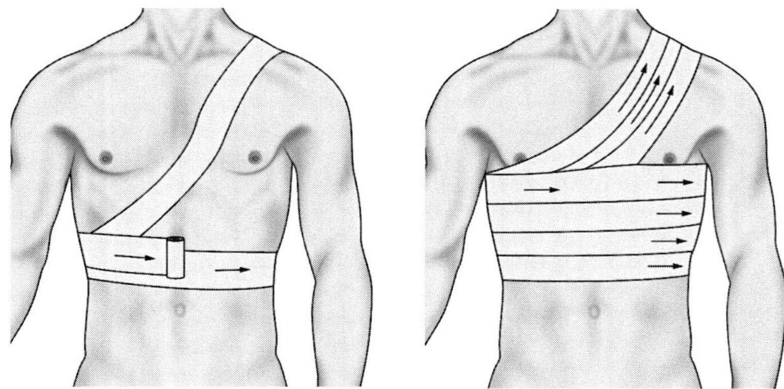

Fig. 13.16: Breast bandage

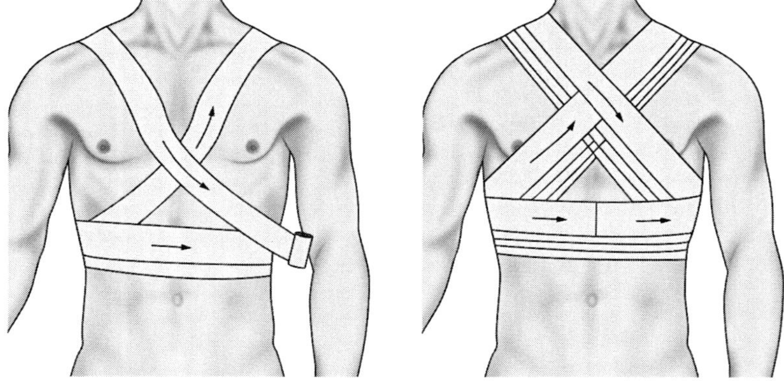

Fig. 13.17: Both breasts bandage

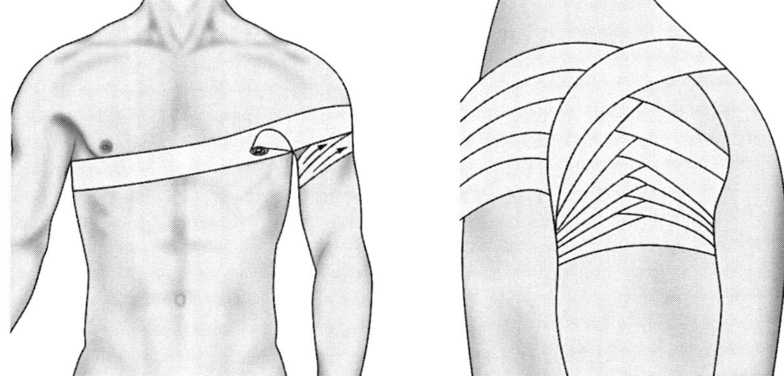

Fig. 13.18: Shoulder spica

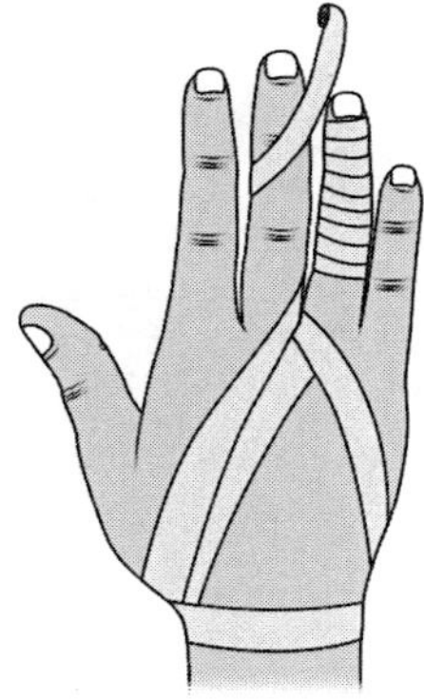

Fig. 13.19: Simple spiral for fingers

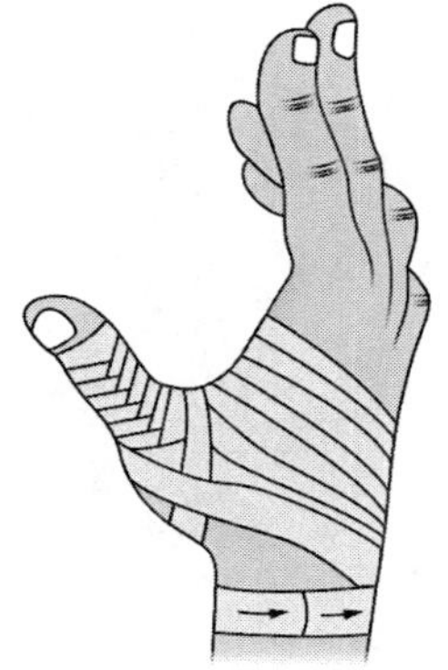

Fig. 13.20: Spica for thumb

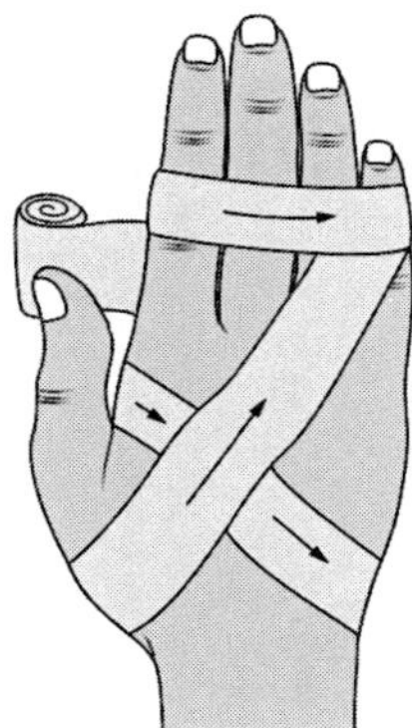

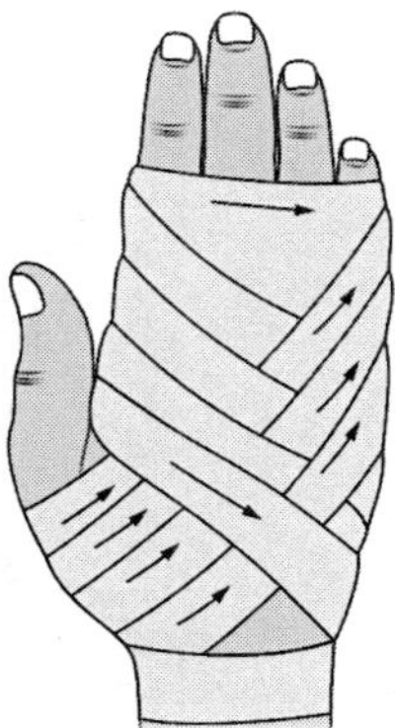

Fig. 13.21: Bandage for hand

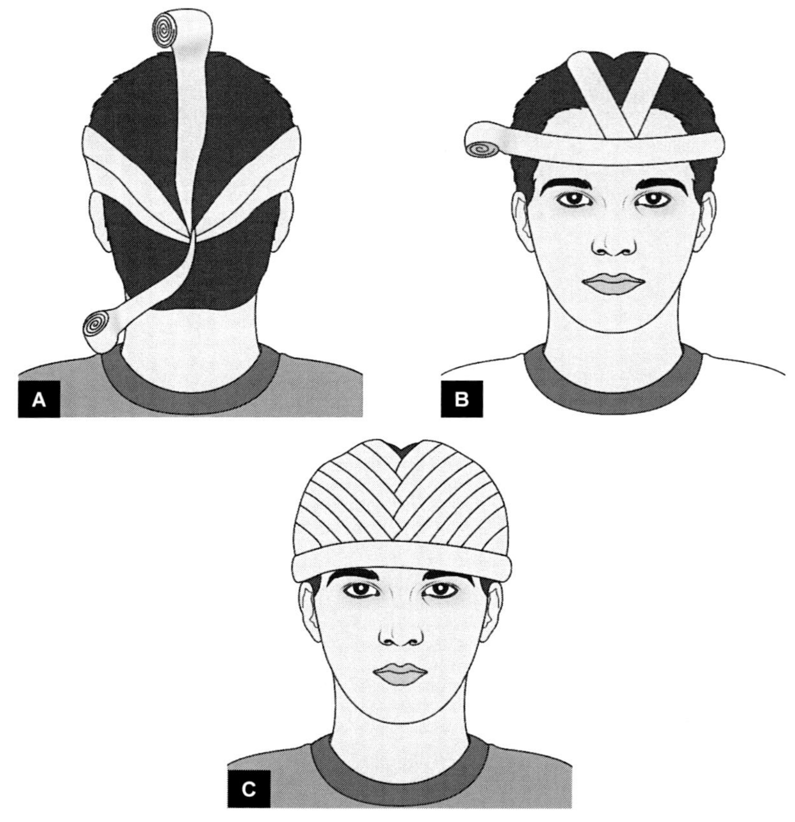

Figs 13.22A to C: Capeline bandage

CHAPTER

14

Meeting Special Needs

AIM

Students are able to care for patients with special needs.

OBJECTIVES

- Students learn care of patients with alterations in body temperature
- Students know the care of patients with alterations in urinary elimination
- Students care for patients with alteration in bowel elimination
- Students learn to care for patients with altered sensorium and sensory deficit
- Students are able to assess self-care ability.

CARE OF PATIENTS WITH ALTERATIONS IN BODY TEMPERATURE

Normal body temperature ranges from 97°F to 99°F. Increase in body temperature is called as fever or pyrexia. It is a sign of disease. Invasion by microorganisms causes fever. It also may be due to viruses. Hot sun in summer causes heat stroke. (see page 79). Fever with chills is rigor. It occurs in malaria, pneumonia, sepsis and urinary tract infections (UTI).

Range of pyrexia:

Low pyrexia—99°F to 101°F.

High pyrexia—101°F to 103° F.

Hyperpyrexia—104°F and above 40°C or more.

Rigor: Fever with Chills

Stages

- **Cold stage:** Patient feels very cold and shivers, stage lasts for 5–10 minutes
- **Hot stage:** Body temperature rises very high from 103°F and above. Patient feels hot. Lips and mucous membrane becomes dry. Skin is hot and dry. This stage lasts for 20–30 minutes
- **Sweating stage:** Patient perspires and body temperature comes down to below normal. This stage lasts for 5–10 minutes. Sometimes, patient may collapse after this stage.

Management

- **Cold stage:** Provide extra warmth by blankets,hot water bag or heating pad,hot drinks like tea, coffee.
- **Hot stage:** Remove blanket. Measures to reduce temperature like putting on fan, cold compress over forehead, ice cap over head. Tepid sponge or cold sponge, cold drinks, juice, ice cream. (see page 81). Check pulse and monitor temperature after 10 minutes
- **Sweating stage:** Wipe dry with towel. Oral care—clean mouth with soda bicarbonate solution, apply glycerine to lips and tongue. Give drugs as ordered. Replace fluids and electrolytes as ordered and measure output and record rigor and output, vitals, general condition of patient. Change clothes, provide comfort and psychological support.
  Hypothermia: see page 78.

CARE OF PATIENTS WITH URINARY ELIMINATION PROBLEMS

- **Incontinence:** Urinary incontinence is involuntary escape of urine that is sufficient to be a problem. It may be temporary or permanent. Leakage of urine may be continuous or intermittent.
  - **Functional:** Involuntary, unpredictable passage of urine in client with intact urinary and nervous system. Urge to void that causes loss of urine before reaching appropriate receptacle
  - **Overflow:** Voluntary or involuntary loss of urine about 20–30 mL from over-distended bladder. Hypotonic or underactive detrusor muscle of bladder, due to drugs, fecal impaction, diabetes, spinal cord injury, enlarged prostate in males and uterine prolapse in females

- **Reflex:** Involuntary loss of urine occurring at somewhat predictable intervals. Large or small amount of urine escapes. It is due to spinal cord dysfunction
- **Stress:** Leakage of small volumes of urine caused by sudden increase in intra-abdominal pressure, e.g. coughing, laughing, sneezing, lifting with full bladder and obesity. Third trimester of pregnancy with uterus in abdomen, incompetent bladder, weak pelvic muscles
- **Urge:** Involuntary passage of urine after strong sense of urgency to void. Decreased bladder capacity, irritation of bladder, stress receptors, use of alcohol or caffeine, increased fluid intake and infection.

Nursing Interventions for Incontinence of Urine

- **Functional:** Habit training, environmental alterations, scheduled toileting, condom catheter for men and protective undergarments
- **Overflow:** Intermittent catheterization, surgery, self-retaining catheter or condom catheter (for males), Crede's method
- **Reflex:** Anticholinergic medicine, surgery, intermittent catheterization, self-retaining catheter or condom catheter for males, estrogen replacement and Crede's method
- **Stress:** Pelvic floor exercises (Kegel), surgery, artificial sphincter, biofeedback, scheduled toileting, electrical stimulation, lifestyle modification, weight reduction exercise
- **Urge:** Anticholinergic drugs, bladder training, treatment of urinary tract infection,vaginitis, lifestyle modifications.

Applying Condom Catheter

Condom catheter is used for males with urinary incontinence. Assess the skin integrity around penis and perineum. Look for signs of skin breakdown, irritation. Assess latex allergy.

Equipment

Condom catheter kit, adhesive strip, urinary drainage bag, disposable gloves, basin with warm water, soap with soap dish, towel and wash cloth.

Explain the procedure to client. Assemble equipment and place at the foot end. Prepare drainage set. Screen the client or close the door. Apply disposable gloves and clean genital area with wash cloth, soap and water. Dry with towel thoroughly. Roll the condom outward onto itself. Hold penis and apply condom by rolling over penis leaving 1–2 inches space between tip of penis and condom. Apply elastic or Velcro strap not too tight or loose. Do not allow elastic or Velcro to come in contact with skin. Connect condom catheter to drainage set. Avoid kinking. Provide comfortable position. Remove equipment and wash hands. Assess client's reaction and document observations made.

CARE OF PATIENTS WITH BOWEL ELIMINATION ALTERATIONS

- **Ostomies:** see page 190
- **Incontinence:** Fecal incontinence is the inability to control passage of feces and gas from the anus. It can harm the client's body image. In many situations, client is mentally alert, but physically not able to avoid defecation. Soiling of clothes can lead to embarrassment and social isolation. Identifying cause is difficult
- **Constipation:** see page 183
- Diarrhea is an increase in number of stools and passage of liquid, unformed feces.

Nursing Interventions

Replacement of fluids and electrolytes, oral and intravenous as ordered. Medication to control diarrhea as ordered. Monitoring vital signs and recording. Preventing shock. Barrier nursing, if infected diarrhea. Send stool for examination.

Bowel Diversions

In some diseases, normal passage of feces through rectum is not possible. Treatment needed for these conditions may require temporary or permanent artificial opening in the abdominal wall called as stoma. If opening is created in ileum, it is called as ileostomy and if in colon, colostomy. Ends of intestine are brought through abdominal wall to create stoma.

- **Continent stoma procedure:**
  - Loop colostomy—These are usually temporary, done in emergency. Large stomas are constructed in transverse colon. Loop of bowel is pulled onto abdominal wall. An external supporting device such as plastic rod, bridge or rubber catheter is temporarily placed under the bowel loop to keep it from slipping back. Bowel is opened and sutured to the skin of abdomen. A communicating wall remains between

proximal and distal bowel. Loop colostomy has two openings through one stoma. The proximal end drains the stool whereas distal portion drains mucus. External supportive device is removed after 7–10 days.
- End colostomy—Stoma is formed from proximal end of the bowel. Distal portion of the gastrointestinal tract is either removed or sewn closed called Hartmann's pouch and left in abdominal cavity. Mainly, it is performed in colorectal cancer where rectum also is removed. Clients with diverticulitis often have temporary end colostomy with Hartmann's pouch
- Double barrel colostomy—Bowel is surgically severed and two ends are brought out onto the abdomen. It has two distinct stomas. Proximal functioning and distal is not functioning

- **Ileoanal pouch anastomosis:** Colon is removed. Pouch is created from the end of the small intestine and is attached to the client's anus. This pouch provides collection of feces which is similar to rectum. The client is continent of stool as stool is evacuated via rectum. When ileorectal pouch is created client has temporary ileostomy to allow anastomosis to heal
- **Kock continent ileostomy:** Small intestine is used to create pouch. The pouch has continent stoma, a nipple like valve that is drained with an external catheter which is placed intermittently in the stoma. Client empties the pouch several times a day. The stoma is covered with a protecting dressing or stoma cap.
- **Colostomy care:**
  - Assist caregiver in selecting appropriate size pouch and skin barrier
  - Inform caregiver the signs of stomal and peristomal skin changes that should be reported
  - Ask caregiver to report characteristics and volume of ostomy output
  - Perform hand hygiene and auscultate bowel sounds
  - Wear gloves. Observe skin barrier and pouch for leakage and length of time in place. Opaque pouch needs removal for observation of stoma whereas clear pouch permits viewing of the stoma without removal
  - Observe stoma for color, swelling, trauma and healing. Stoma should be moist and reddish pink
  - Measure the stoma with each pouching change
  - Observe abdominal incision, if present
  - After removing skin barrier and pouch, assess skin around stoma noting scars,folds,skin breakdowns, peristomal suture line, if present. Keep pouch loosely attached to stoma to collect any drainage while system is being changed

- Determine client's emotional response and knowledge and understanding of an ostomy and its care
- Explain procedure to client and get cooperation
- Perform hand hygiene and wear disposable gloves
- Place towel or disposable waterproof barrier under the client. Completely remove skin barrier and pouch pushing back the skin away from barrier. Adhesive remover may be used
- Clean peristomal skin gently with warm water using gauze or washcloth. Do not scrub, dry completely by patting the skin with gauze or towel
- Measure the stoma for correct size of pouching system needed. Prepare pouch by removing backing from barrier and adhesive. Apply thin circle of barrier paste around opening in pouch. Allow it to dry
- Apply the skin barrier and pouch (Fig. 14.1). If creases next to stoma occur, use barrier paste to fill in. Let it dry for 1–2 minutes
- Ostomy deodorant is sometimes used into pouch
- Fold bottom of open-ended pouches up once and close using a closure device such as clamp
- Properly dispose of old pouch and soiled equipment. Spray deodorant in room, if needed.

CARE OF PATIENTS WITH PROBLEMS OF SENSORIUM (TABLE 14.1)

In certain conditions sensory and motor function is disturbed causing paraplegia, hemiplegia and unconsciousness.

Paraplegia is a condition where patient has paralysis of lower limbs. Injury or compression of spinal cord causes loss of sensory and motor functions. Patient loses control over bladder and bowel.

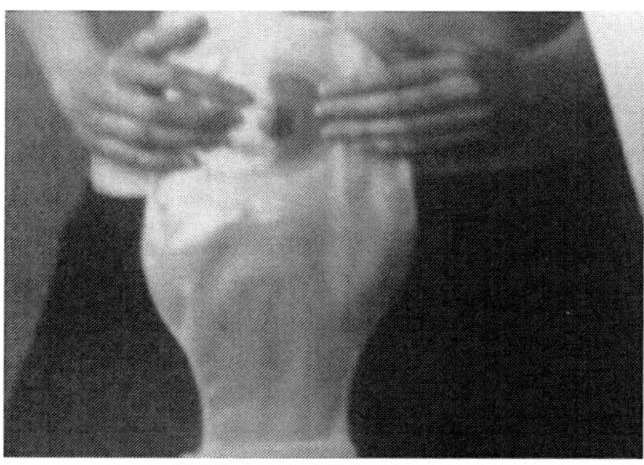

Fig. 14.1: Colostomy pouch applied over stoma

Management

Table 14.1: Management of patients with problems of sensorium

Nursing diagnosis	*Nursing interventions*
Risk of developing pressure ulcers r/to loss of sensation, immobility, incontinence Risk of developing foot drop r/to paralysis of lower limbs Self-care deficit Bowel incontinence Need for nutrition Immobility Risk for developing infection through continued use of self-retaining catheter	Change of position every two hours Change of position every two hours Back rub every four hours Condom catheter for males and self-retaining catheter to females Keep the bed clean and dry Passive exercise of lower limbs Use of extra pillows Foot support 'Splinting' of limb Daily bed bath, oral care, assistance, hair care. Providing bedpan at regular interval for bowel training Full diet with vitamin supplements. Vitamin B1, B6, B12 containing food Passive exercise, range of movements, massage to back and lower limbs Releasing catheter every 4 hours instead of continuous drainage and bladder training

r/to, resulting to

Care of Patients with Hemiplegia (Table 14.2)

Hemiplegia is a condition where patient has loss of sensory and motor functions of one side of the body either left or right. Condition is usually due to stroke.

Management

Table 14.2: Management of patients with hemiplegia

Nursing diagnosis	*Nursing intervention*
Risk of developing pressure ulcers, r/to loss of sensation, immobility, incontinence Self-care deficit Need for nutrition Immobility Risk for aspiration, facial paralysis Aphasia Bowel control deficit Stress incontinence Risk for eye infection and dryness of cornea	Change of position every two hours Backrub every four hours Condom catheter for males and self-retaining catheter to females Keep the bed clean and dry Passive exercise of lower limbs Use of extra pillows Daily bed bath, oral care assistance, hair care Providing bedpan at regular interval for bowel training

Contd...

Nursing diagnosis	*Nursing intervention*
Depression r/to sudden loss of sensation, movements, absence from job, less hope of recovery	Full diet with vitamin supplements. Vitamin B1, B6, B12 containing food Range of movement hand and legs, body massage Suction of pharynx, as needed Observe nonverbal communication Provide call bell, paper and pen Bowel training. Providing bedpan at regular interval Condom catheter for males Bladder training Instill eye drops as ordered Psychological support, counseling by expert Physiotherapy, occupational therapy, social support, referring to social organizations for support Need for rehabilitation

Care of Unconscious Patients

Unconsciousness is loss of sensory and motor functions. It may be due to cerebral hemorrhage, head injury, drugs, poisoning, diabetic coma, uremic coma, hyperpyrexia, excessive alcohol, after convulsions, eclampsia, hepatic coma. Consciousness may come after treatment of cause.

Management

- Safety
- Keeping airway patent
- Monitoring vital signs
- Eye care
- Oral care
- Preventing pressure ulcers
- Nutrition
- Care of bladder and bowels
- Preventing respiratory infection
- Personal hygiene.

Patients are kept in intensive care unit. Patient is kept in comfortable bed with railings on both sides water mattress protected with full mackintosh. Airway is kept patent with airway in mouth. Frequent suctioning is done to prevent oral secretions entering respiratory tract. Instill eye drops as ordered to prevent corneal dryness. Eyes are cleaned everyday when giving bed bath. Oral care is given every four hours. Mouth is cleaned with soda bicarbonate solution and glycerine is applied over lips and tongue. Ryle's tube feeding is given. Nutritious liquids like milk, fruit juice, soup, fortified liquids are given. IV fluids for elecrocyte balance. Self-retaining catheter is put in bladder and urobag is connected for collecting and measuring output. Specimens are sent for investigations. Condom catheter is applied for males. Antibiotics are given as ordered. Position is changed every two hours. Left lateral, right lateral, three-fourth prone positions are used with extra pillows for support. Back rub is given every four hours and observation of skin at pressure points is done and record. Vital signs are monitored continuously. Daily bed bath, change of clothes. Keeping bed linen clean and dry. Movements of limbs and chest physiotherapy. Ventilatory support, when needed. Intermittent oxygen therapy.

CARE OF PATIENTS IN SHOCK

Shock results from failure of cardiovascular system to provide sufficient blood circulation, oxygen to all parts of the body.

Causes

- Severe loss of blood, body fluids
- Intense pain
- Excessive trauma
- Burns
- Poisoning
- Emotional stress
- Extreme heat or cold
- Allergic reaction
- Sudden or severe illness
- Severe infection.

Types

- **Hypovolemic shock:** It occurs due to blood loss, fluid volume loss in vomiting and diarrhea
- **Cardiogenic shock:** It results from poor cardiac function
- **Neurogenic shock:** It is due to nervous system not able to contract blood vessels
- **Septic shock:** It results from severe infection, microbes causing escape of fluid from blood vessels
- **Psychogenic shock:** It is caused due to emotional response to external stimuli

- **Anaphylactic shock:** It is due to sudden severe reaction of body to allergens. In condition of shock, there is sudden lowering of blood pressure, fast and thready pulse which is not felt later on, air hunger. Patient may become unconscious. Cyanosis is present. Skin is cold, clammy and sweating. Tremors may be seen.

Management

Preventing shock before it is established. Control of hemorrhage, fluid replacement in cases of diarrhea, vomiting, burns, high fevers.

Maintaining patent airway and oxygen therapy. Keep head to one side till airway is introduced. Replacement of fluids. Start IV line with dextrose 5%. Give drugs as ordered. Replacing fluids dextrose, normal saline, ringer lactate. Arrange for blood. Send blood for grouping and cross matching. Start blood immediately as ordered. Monitor vital signs every 15 minutes till patient recovers. Head low position.

Sensory Impairment

Most common types of sensory impairment are sensory deficit, sensory deprivation and sensory overload. Ability to function and relate effectively with the environment is seriously impaired.

Sensory Deficit

A deficit in normal sensory reception and perception. When senses are impaired, sense of self is impaired. Person avoids communication or mixing with others. Person relies on unaffected senses. Some senses may become acute to compensate.

Sensory Deprivation

When a person experiences an adequate quality and quantity of stimulation, sensory deprivation occurs. For ego patient admitted in intensive care unit is deprived of other external stimuli, except technical interventions.

Sensory Overload

When person receives multiple sensory stimuli overload occurs. Client in constant pain or frequently monitored vital signs, irritation from drainage, wound has sensory overload. Behavioral changes associated with overload can be confusion, disorientation, restlessness and anxiety. Clients in intensive care unit sometimes resort to constantly fingering tubes and dressing.

Common Sensory Deficits

- **Visual deficit:** Presbyopia, cataract, dry eyes, glaucoma, retinopathy, macular degeneration can cause visual deficit
- **Hearing deficit:** Presbycusis is progressive hearing disorder of old age. Cerumen accumulation can cause hearing deficit
- **Balance deficit:** Dizziness and disequilibrium is common condition resulting from vestibular dysfunction
- **Taste deficit:** Xerostomia is decrease in salivation leading to dry mouth
- **Neurological deficit:** Peripheral neuropathy commonly found in diabetic patients, Guillain-Barre syndrome, neoplasms causing tingling and numbness of affected area and stumbling gait.

Stroke

Cerebrovascular accident caused by clot, hemorrhage or emboli, obstructing blood flow to the brain creates incoordination and imbalance, loss of sensation of limbs. Loss of motor activities of limbs. If left hemisphere is affected, difficulty in speech may occur.

Factors Affecting Sensory Functions

Age

Infants are not able to discriminate sensory stimuli. Presbyopia needs glasses for reading at the age of 40 years and above. Aging reduces visual field, increased glare sensitivity, impaired night vision, reduced accommodation and color discrimination. Hearing changes beginning at the age of 30 years decreasing acuity, pitch discrimination, hearing threshold. Proprioceptive changes after 60 years of age include difficulty in balance, spatial orientation, coordination. Older adults experience tactile changes including declining sensitivity to pain, pressure and temperature.

Assessing Self-care Ability

Nurse assesses client's functional abilities in their home environment or hospital for feeding, dressing, grooming and toileting activities. Asses for loss of balance in toileting, assess, if client can see items in feeding tray, reading paper, writing cheque, reading bills, etc. Assess, if client can perform those activities of daily living by asking them to do and observing. If not, assisting with these activities.

CHAPTER

15

Care of Terminally Ill Patient

AIM

Students care for terminally ill patients.

OBJECTIVES

- Students know the concept of loss and grief
- Student know hospice care
- Students know care after death and medicolegal issues.

CONCEPT OF LOSS

Losses are integral part of individual's life. We expect our losses to be recovered and replaced by something better. Losses that cause us to suffer or unbearable change, which can not be recovered like death of loved one, divorce, loss of independence are significant and give long-term effect on health. Person experiences loss in absence of object, person, body part, function, emotion or idea that was previously present. Loss may be actual or perceived. Actual loss is any loss of person or object that can no longer be felt or heard, known or experienced by an individual. Perceived loss is the loss of confidence, and prestige. Loss may be maturational or situational. Maturational loss is any change in the developmental process normally expected. Situational loss is any sudden, unexpected external event, e.g. accident. Death is ultimate loss. It is mystical event that creates anxiety and fear. Death ends relationship that binds and unites family and individual.

GRIEF AND GRIEVING PROCESS

Grief is emotional response to loss. Coping with grief after loss involves the process of mourning, outward expression of loss. It involves working through the grief until an individual adapts to his or her expectations to go on in life without that which was lost. Inner feelings and outward reactions of the survivor are grieving and mourning, together called as bereavement. Individual may move back and forth through series of stages, extending for period of years. No one gets over loss but the individual can heal and learn to live with loss.

Kubler Ross's five stages: Denial, anger, bargaining, depression and acceptance.

Bowlby's four phases: Numbing, yearning and search, disorganization and despair, reorganization.

Worden's four stages: To accept reality of loss, to work through pain of grief, to adjust to an environment, emotionally relocate and move on with life.

HOSPICE CARE

The concept of hospice is that of a caring community of professional and nonprofessional people, together with family. Emphasis as on dealing with emotional and spiritual problems as well as the medical problems of terminally ill patients.

Of primary concern is control of pain and other symptoms, keeping the patient at home for as long as possible or desirable and making the remaining days as comfortable and meaningful as possible. After the patient dies, family members are given support throughout their period of bereavement.

Generally clients accepted into hospice program have less than six months to live. Hospice services are available in the home, hospital and nursing home settings.

Components of Hospice Care

Client and family as a unit of care. Home care with inpatient beds. Control of symptoms. Physician directed services. Care by doctors, nurses, social workers, counselors and spiritual advisors. Medical and nursing services are available all the time. Many clients prefer to die at home in familiar setting whereas others choose not to burden their families. There must be primary care offered at home.

There is always an effort to keep the client at home for as long as possible. The family provides basic supportive care. Home care aid is always available and nurse is available to coordinate and administer symptom management therapies. Twenty-four hours interdisciplinary accessibility as needed. As client's death becomes imminent, members of hospice team are present to give support to client and family.

Signs of Approaching Death

Refuses food and drinks, urinary output reduced, sleep, impaired vision and hearing, speech difficult to understand, secretions collected at back of throat, rattle or gurgle, irregular breathing or apnea, restlessness, hot and cold feeling alternately, loss of bladder bowel control, see many things like garden, libraries, dead persons, may ask for packing of luggage, passport ticket, etc. hazy cornea, lowering of vital signs, hypothermia, sluggish reflexes, loss of muscle tone, dehydration or fluids escaping from opened body sphincters.

Care of Dying Patient

Nurse promotes client's self-esteem and dignity. Maintains strengthening, empathic and therapeutic communication. Spends time to let client share their life experiences and provide spiritual comfort.

Attend to client's appearance and surroundings, cleanliness, absence of body odors, attractive clothing, personal grooming to contribute to sense of worth. Client is often fearful of dying alone, it is important to attend call light quickly.

Perform assessment and use appropriate touch when caring. Clients can share companionship and conversation in group. When family members come, talk to them and keep them informed about client's progress. Give hints what to discuss with client. Ask family members to perform simple activities of care. Allow visitors to remain with patient. Know the ways and means to contact family members at any time, if client requests or condition worsens.

Frequent repositioning, keeping bedlinen dry, controlling noise, showing of cherishing pictures, objects, cards, letters, soft music, pleasant environment will help to sleep and minimize severity of symptoms.

Skin care: Bath, skin lubricants, clean and dry bed linen, change position.

Oral care: 2–4 hourly. Use soft toothbrush. Apply glycerine or vaseline to lips, glycerine to tongue.

Eye care: Remove crust with wet swab, artificial tears to reduce corneal drying.
Rest: Promote rest and provide quiet environment, time and pace nursing activities.
Diet: Liquids frequently, bran, soup, low residue diet, home cooked foods. stool softeners.
Condom drainage or indwelling catheter.

Signs of Clinical Death

Death: The cessation of all physical and chemical processes that occur in all the living organisms or their cellular components. Absence of heart beat and cessation of breathing is clinical death.
Brain death: Performance of brain death criteria under the appropriate circumstances allows the patient a dignified death, reduces the agony of the relatives and releases the scarce resources for other seriously ill patients.

Death Certificate

Certificate issued by the registrar for death after receipt of preliminary certificate completed and signed by an attending doctor indicating date, time, and probable cause of death.

Advance Directives

There are two basic advance directives.

1. Living wills.
2. Durable powers of attorney for health care.

Living Wills

Living wills are written documents that direct treatment in accordance with the client's wishes in the event of terminal illness or condition. Living will may be difficult to interpret and not clinically specific in unforeseen circumstances. Two witnesses, excluding physician and relatives are needed.

Durable Power of Attorney for Health Care

Designates an agent, surrogate or proxy to make health care decisions if and when the client is no longer able to make decisions on his or her own behalf.

Organ Donation

For transplantation of organs, client must be maintained on ventilator and circulatory support until vital organs are harvested. Family must clearly understand that the client is brain dead, that the ventilator and the medication is not keeping the client alive but keeping the physical body in a state so that organs will not be damaged. Organ, tissue donation must be agreed by the family if no specific document is made by client before death.

Dying Declaration

It is declaration of will by dying patient. It should be written and signed by two witnesses. It is valid in the court of law.

Medicolegal Issues

Death is informed to police, if it is medicolegal and body is sent for postmortem examination.

Last Offices

It is important that in postmortem care nurse cares for client's body with dignity and sensitivity. After death body undergoes many physical changes. For that reason, care must be provided immediately to prevent damage and disfigurement. Client must be maintained on ventilatory and circulatory support until vital organs are harvested even after client is pronounced dead. If organ retrieval is to be done, legal process should be carried out.

Care after Death

Equipment

Bath towels, washcloths, washbasin, scissors, name tags, bed linen, and room deodorizer, documentation forms.

- Physician must certify death
- Autopsy, organs for donation, if opted, required procedure is to be done
- If body is to be sent for postmortem check the order
- Remove all equipment, tubes, supplies, dirty linen and screen the patient
- Cleanse body thoroughly, apply clean sheet and remove all trash from room
- Brush and comb hair.

- Close eyes gently, pack openings of body, wrap till neck, and tie hands, feet
- Put label—Contact number, name, age, sex, register number, date and time of death, diagnosis, one on wrist, one on right toe, and one outside the shroud
- Wash hands
- Complete documentation on nurses notes
- Clarify personal belongings that are to stay with body or document who has taken personal items, time, date, sign of receiver
- Disinfection of linen, equipment, disposal of articles, after caring for, if patient is suffering from communicable disease, special precautions are to be taken. Wear mask, gown, and gloves.

Autopsy

Postmortem examination of body to determine the cause of death. Some body parts specimens are sent for laboratory study. Postmortem examination is done by experienced authorized medical officer and provides report for medical record and in the court of law.

Embalming

Injection of formalin in to various body tissues to prevent disintegration for few days. The procedure is done in specialized department of medical college and hospital usually government medical college and civil hospital.

CHAPTER

16

Professional Nursing: Concepts and Practice

AIM

Students are oriented with theories and models of nursing.

OBJECTIVES

- Students know various theories of nursing
- Students know models of nursing
- Students know concepts of nursing and practice.

CONCEPTUAL AND THEORETICAL MODELS OF NURSING

Theories and models of nursing are concepts, definitions, relationships generating knowledge to apply in nursing practice. Application of nursing process in practice is a result of various theories and models. Concept maps, critical paths and care plans are prepared for nursing practice on the basis of nursing theories and models. When caring for clients they are considered as person with various aspects. Basic facts in all theories and models consists of patient, environment, health and nursing care which enable us to give patient care.

INTRODUCTION TO MODELS

Model refers to global ideas about the group, individual, situation or event.

Holistic Model

Holistic model considers patient as whole. Person is whole with various cells, tissues, organs, systems functioning harmoniously with its physiological and spiritual aspect. When treatment is given or surgery is performed, it is not only related to part of the body but it affects patient as a whole. Uderstanding patient as a person is necessary in finding out his lifestyle, his strengths and weaknesses, his resource, heredity, social and family background, diet, religious facts, thinking, attitude towads life and philosophy of life, for the diagnosis, treatment and health education. Person has various needs—physical, psychological, social, spiritual, and personal motives which in turn affect a person. To understand these needs and provide care understanding patient as a person is necessary.

Health Belief Model

Rosenstoch's and Becker health belief model: Model shows relationship between a person's beliefs and behavior. It gives idea about way of understanding and behavior of clients in relation to their health and how they will comply with healthcare therapies.

Components

- Individual's perception of susceptibility to illness
- Individual's perception of seriousness of the illness
- Likelihood that a person will take preventive action.

Health belief model helps nurses to understand factors influencing client's perception, beliefs and behavior in order to plan effective care.

INTRODUCTION TO THEORIES IN NURSING

Theory is a set of concepts, definitions, relationship and assumptions which explain systematic phenomenon. Nursing theory consists of some aspects of nursing explained, predicted and nursing care is prescribed. Nursing theories make nurses to view client's situation, organize data, analyze and interpret. Application of nursing theory in practice depends on nurse's knowledge of nursing, theoretical model, their relationship and use of those in designing nursing interventions.

Concept

Concepts are mental images of an object or event depending on individual's perception. Concepts may be of various aspects.

Definitions

It gives general meaning of the concept that fits into theory.

Assumption

Assumptions are statements that describe concepts or connect two concepts that are factual.

Phenomenon

Phenomenon is aspect of reality that can be experienced. For example, self-care, response to stress.

Types of Theories

Grand theories, middle range theories, descriptive theories and prescriptive theories.

Linking Theories with Nursing Process

Theories generate nursing knowledge which is used in nursing practice. Integrating theory with nursing practice is the basis of professional nursing. Nursing process is used in practice. Components of nursing process like making nursing diagnosis requires analysis and critical thinking. It is scientific process of collecting data, analyzing and interpreting, which are similar to components of theory. In nursing theory, concepts are defined, projected, supported by data, analyzed and interpreted but it is at very large scale or in depth. Theory is knowledge whereas nursing process is application in practice.

Florence Nightingale's Theory

She did not view nursing as limited to administration of medicine and treatment, but it is oriented towards providing fresh air, light, warmth, cleanliness, quiet and adequate nutrition.

Henderson's Theory

Henderson defines nursing as individual sick or well, assisting in those activities that will contribute to health, recovery or peaceful death, and that the individual would perform unaided, if he or she had necessary strength, will or knowledge. The process of nursing tries to do this as rapidly as possible and the goal is independence.

Henderson's 14 basicneeds: Physiological, psychological, sociocultural, spiritual and developmental.

BETTY-NEUMAN'S MODEL

He defines total person model of nursing, incorporating holistic concept and an open system approach. Nursing is concerned with whole person. Goal of nursing is to assist individual, families, groups in attaining and maintaining a maximum level of total wellness. The nurse assesses, manages, evaluates client's systems. Nursing focuses on the variables affecting the client's response to the stressors. Nursing actions include primary, secondary and tertiary levels of prevention. Primary prevention—strengthening line of defense by identifying risk factors, stressors. Secondary prevention—strengthening internal defense and resources—establishing priorities, treatment plans. Tertiary prevention—readaptation, strengthening resistance to stressors and assisting in prevention of recurrence.

DOROTHEA OREM: SELF-CARE MODEL

It is learned, goal-oriented activity directed towards the self in the interest of maintaining life, health, development and well-being. Help client to perform self-care. Assess self-care needs, deficits, abilities. Design individualized nursing interventions.

ROY'S THEORY

Sister Callista Roy: Adaptation theory—she views client as adaptive system. Goal of nursing is to help the person adapt to changes in physiological needs, self-concepts, role functions and independent relation during health and illness. Meeting basic physiological needs, developing positive self-concept, performing social roles, achieving balance between dependence and independence.

MARTHA ROGER'S THEORY

It focuses on person's wholeness. Seek to promote symphonic interactions between two energy fields—human and environmental. Coordinate the human field with rhythmicity of the environmental fields. Direct pattern of interactions and redirect interventions between two energy fields to promote maximum health potential.

LINKING THEORY WITH NURSING PROCESS

Theories and models are result of many years study, experience, based on observations, collection of data, analyzing and interpreting. Nursing process is implementation of theory in practice. Holistic model, self-care model, environmental model are all used in practice through nursing process, i.e identifying problems, needs of patient prioritization planning and implementing, evaluating and replaning.

Utilizing theories and models in practice, i.e. patient care, providing conducive environment, lifesaving procedures and preventive measures. Using different principles in practice to protect self and others and for the social good.

Index

Page numbers followed by *f* refer to figure and *t* refer to table.

C

G

H

I

N

U

V

W